Our Greatest Threats: Live Longer, Live Better

William M. Manger, MD, PhD

Founder and Chairman,
National Hypertension Association
Founder and Director, VITAL
(Values Initiative Teaching About Lifestyle)
Clinical Professor of Medicine, NYU Medical Center
Emeritus Lecturer in Medicine,
Columbia Medical School
Designated Distinguished Mayo Alumnus

JONES AND BARTLETT PUBLISHERS
Sudbury, Massachusetts
BOSTON TORONTO LONDON SINGAPORE

World Headquarters
Jones and Bartlett
Publishers
40 Tall Pine Drive
Sudbury, MA 01776
978-443-5000
info@jbpub.com
www.jbpub.com

Jones and Bartlett
Publishers
Canada
6339 Ormindale Way
Mississauga, Ontario
L5V 1J2
CANADA

Jones and Bartlett
Publishers
International
Barb House, Barb M7ews
London W6 7PA
UK

Jones and Bartlett's books and products are available through most bookstores and on-line booksellers. To contact Jones and Bartlett Publishers directly, call 800-832-0034, fax 978-443-8000, or visit our website, www.jbpub.com.

Substantial discounts on bulk quantities of Jones and Bartlett's publications are available to corporations, professional associations, and other qualified organizations. For details and specific discount information, contact the special sales department at Jones and Bartlett via the above contact information or send an email to specialsales@jbpub.com.

Copyright © 2006 by William M. Manger, MD, PhD.

LIBRARY OF CONGRESS CATALOGING-IN-PUBLICATION DATA
Manger, William Muir, 1920-
    Our greatest threats : live longer, live better / William M. Manger.
      p. cm.
    Includes bibliographical references and index.
    ISBN 0-7637-3944-8 (pbk.)
    1. Longevity. 2. Health. 3. Self-care, Health. I. Title.
    RA776.75.M362 2005
    613.2--dc22
                                 2005023422

PRODUCTION CREDITS
Executive Publisher: Christopher Davis
Associate Editor: Kathy Richardson
Production Director: Amy Rose
Associate Production Editor: Kate Hennessy
Associate Marketing Manager: Laura Kavigian
V.P. Manufacturing and Inventory Control: Therese Connell
Composition: Pageworks
Cover Concept: Victoria Hartman, William M. Manger
Cover Layout: Timothy Dziewit
Senior Photo Researcher: Kimberly Potvin
Printing and Binding: Malloy, Inc.
Cover Printing: Malloy, Inc.
Additional photo credits appear on page 252,
    which constitutes a continuation of the copyright page.

Printed in the United States of America
09 08 07 06 05   10 9 8 7 6 5 4 3 2 1

- Live safer
- Live healthier
- Live longer
- Feel better
- Look better
- Work better
- Play better
- Sleep better
- Improve your self-esteem
- Improve your quality of life
- Increase your energy
- Enjoy better sex
- Reduce stress
- Be happier

This includes a section on the DASH diet, recommended by the American Heart Association, the National Cancer Institute, the National High Blood Pressure Education Program, and Medical Profession and Nutritionists as the best diet for reducing elevated blood pressure and maintaining health; with appropriate modifications, it is an excellent diet to treat diabetes, lower blood fats, and reduce weight! A DASH food pyramid is included.

Ten important factors that can impact your health and lifestyle

1. Nutrition
2. Exercise
3. Salt
4. Alcohol
5. Cigarettes
6. Drugs
7. Sleep
8. Sex
9. Safety
10. Stress

Dedication

To my grandchildren—Samantha, Catherine, and Jackson—
and for all of those children and adults who improve their
lifestyle and strengthen the health of our nation.

Contents

Preface   xv
Foreword I   xvii
Foreword II   xix
Foreword III   xxi
Foreword IV   xxiii
Foreword V   xxvii

Section I   Introduction   **1**

You can change your lifestyle
Overeating
Toxic food and beverage environment
Motivation
Prevention by healthy lifestyle

Section II   Overweight and Obesity Crisis   **9**

Major threat to our nation
Simple determination of approximate ideal weight
Body Mass Index (BMI)
Fast foods and obesity
Health consequences of obesity
"The Deadly Quartet"
Selecting a healthy diet
Dangers of some dietary supplements

Section III   The Best Eating Plan   **35**

Definition of the best diet
Avoid foods containing cholesterol and harmful fats

Limit simple carbohydrates, foods high in sugar
Increase dietary fiber
Consume adequate vitamins and minerals
Limit saturated fat, trans-fat
Do not change percent of dietary protein
The DASH diet and its benefits
Butter substitutes
Good strategies for healthy eating
Foods to choose or limit
Tips on losing weight
Atkins, Ornish, Pritikin, Agatston ("South Beach"), Sears
    ("Zone"), and Steward ("Sugar Busters") Diets
Food groups, examples, and calories

Section IV   Risks of Salt   67

Table salt (sodium chloride) and hypertension
Recommended daily dietary sodium
Salt substitutes
Salt and water consumption by marathon runners
Foods high in sodium content

**Section V   Physical Activity and Exercise—Risks of
    Inactivity**   75

Sedentary lifestyle of Americans
Overuse of TV and computers
Obesity in children
Consequences of sedentary lifestyle
Benefits of regular aerobic exercise
Recommended physical activity and calories burned

Section VI   Risks of Alcohol   85

Alcohol, the drug of choice among teenagers
Main cause of fatal teenage car injuries

Consequences of chronic alcoholism
Alcohol and hypertension
Caloric content of alcohol
Cessation of alcohol consumption
Interaction of alcohol and drugs

Section VII   Risks of Cigarette Smoking   **93**

Harmful effects of cigarette smoking
Effect of nicotine in cigarettes
Risks of "passive smoking"
Teenage smokers
Importance of smoking prevention and cessation
Hazards of smokeless tobacco

Section VIII   How to Quit Smoking   **103**

Importance of motivation (desire) to quit
It's never too late to quit
Suggestions and approaches to smoking cessation

**Section IX   Risks of Using Illicit and Some
Prescription Drugs**   **109**

Effects of marijuana:
    Harmful effects, contamination, mood alterations
    Automobile injuries
    Development of tolerance
    Concerns over legalization
Effects of hallucinogens:
    LSD
    Mescaline
    Phencyclidine
    Psilocybin
Effects of stimulants:
    Amphetamine

    Methamphetamine

    Cocaine, Crack, and Crank

    Ecstasy

    Khat

    Betel nuts

Effects of inhalants:

    Dangers of common inhalants (particularly popular with
        children and teenagers)

    Amyl nitrite

    Whippet

Effects of sedatives:

    Ketamine (date rape drug)

    GHB (date rape drug)

    Rohypnol (date rape drug)

    Klonopin

    Barbiturates

    Quaaludes

Opiates or opiate-like substances

    Opium, Morphine, Heroin, Codeine,
        Dextromethorphan, Methadone

    Heroin addicts

    Signs and symptoms of drug use

    Detoxification

Steroids, Creatine, and DHEAs (dehydroepiandrosterone
    sulfate)

    Use and harmful effects of steroids

    Use of creatine to build muscle mass

    Use of DHEAs to build muscle mass and its harmful
        effects

Effects and complications caused by illicit drugs

Illicit drugs and alcohol use in teenagers

Recognition of illicit drug and alcohol use

Treatment, rehabilitation, and support programs

A practical parenting guide to deal with children using
    illicit drugs

Section X   Risks of Sexually Transmitted Disease   *127*

> Magnitude of AIDS and HIV infection in USA
> Curable and incurable STDs
> Emphasis of sex education and prevention
> Prevalence of teenage pregnancy
> Importance of latex condom in STD prevention
> Conditions increasing risk of HIV infection
> Abstinence guarantees safety from STDs and pregnancy

Section XI   Safety Measures to Prevent Injuries and
*   Some Diseases*   *133*

> Safety on the road:
>   Automobiles
>   Precautions for other types of transportation and
>   recreation
>   Pedestrians
> Safety on or in the water:
>   Boating
>   Swimming, diving, and surfing
>   Shark attacks
>   Swimming pools
>   Contaminated water
> Safety in the sun:
>   Sunburn
>   Malignant melanoma
> Safety at home:
>   Fire
>   Carbon monoxide
>   Gas leak and fumes
>   Knives and sharp instruments
>   Window bars and safety gates
>   Tools and machinery
>   Pistols and guns
>   Electric shock

Safe food preparation
Safety of children:
    Toy safety and suffocation
    Clothing
    Pedophiles
Safety of elderly:
    Falls
    Sensitivity to heat and cold
    Living alone
Environmental hazards:
    Poisonings
    Mercury
    Lead
    Asbestos
    Arsenic
    Mold/fungi
Weather-related hazards:
    Lightning
    Hurricanes/floods
    Tornadoes
    Earthquakes/tsunamis
    Cold weather
Homeland security and terrorism
Avoiding bites:
    Rabies
    Insects
    Snakes
    Scorpions
    Ticks
    Lyme disease
Avoiding bear attacks
Health emergencies:
    Blood clots
    Heart attacks
    Strokes

Preventive measures for your health:
    Immunization
    Eye and ear safety
    Health screenings
    Minimizing health care errors
First aid courses:
    CPR
    Heimlich maneuvers

Section XII   Risks of Inadequate Sleep   **211**

    Consequences of sleep deprivation
    Hours of sleep recommended for adults and children
    Sleep apnea
    Ensuring children get adequate sleep
    Medications and conditions that may disrupt sleep

Section XIII   Stress Risks   **217**

    Factors contributing to chronic stress

Section XIV   Concluding Remarks   **221**

    Importance of recognizing different abilities
    Importance of encouragement
    Importance of a healthy lifestyle
    VITAL (Values Initiative Teaching About Lifestyle)
    Key to healthy lifestyle—prevention

Acknowledgments   225

Commentaries   229

Index   239

Author Biography   251

Our nation was built primarily on "family, faith, and hard work"; furthermore, the remarkable success of this democracy depends, to a very large extent, on the freedom we all enjoy so much. People in all parts of the world desire and seek freedom as a central ingredient of happiness. However, most would agree that **freedom without responsibility is unworkable and can only eventually lead to decadence and deterioration of any society.** My late brother, Jules Manger, used to say that to complement the Statue of Liberty on the East Coast we should also have a Statue of Responsibility on the West Coast of the United States. In my opinion, his suggestion was right on target because **we all should appreciate, more than ever, the crucial role of responsibility in our lives and the lives of our children.**

Within only the past few decades, there are increasing signs that responsibility, in a variety of areas, is not a major concern of many Americans. Erosion of belief in values and responsibility can undermine and sap the strength and health of our nation. We face a very serious health crisis involving diseases that result from unhealthy lifestyles. Health care for these diseases has created an enormous financial burden on the public and the government of this nation. It is essential that we all work together to stem and prevent this medical crisis, which continues to increase. The importance of healthy lifestyles to preserve the health of Americans has never been more evident. The purpose of *Our Greatest Threats* is to encourage, educate, and empower adults and children to seek a healthier and safer lifestyle.

This book addresses the very core of our well-being—namely, our lifestyle. The basic and vital information and recommendations in this book will provide important guidance for those interested in improving their health and safety and that of their family. **Success by adherence to a healthy lifestyle depends on persistent motivation, which, of course, is up to you.**

Case reports are included to illustrate some of the devastating consequences of unhealthy lifestyles. The accounts are fairly accurate, but to observe privacy, only the initials of individuals are used. However, in one case, the identity of the individual is revealed, as the occurrence of a massive and fatal stroke in the 32nd President of the United States is well-documented and public knowledge. The progressive development of his hypertension (high blood pressure) was probably not the result of an unhealthy lifestyle, but was due to the absence of any antihypertensive medication at the time.

Francis Bacon said, "Some books are to be tasted, others to be swallowed, and some few to be chewed and digested." I pray that this book is worthy of the latter category!

William M. Manger, MD, PhD

"May you and all of us be enabled to lead our young people along a better, more noble path."

The Late Cannon Charles Martin
Reverend and Beloved Headmaster of St. Alban's School

Dr. William Manger's remarkable new book, *Our Greatest Threats,* is a tool of immeasurable service to all adults who care for and about children. For many years, Dr. Manger has been active in urging Americans to embrace a lifestyle that emphasizes exercise and diet in order to develop health, energy, and pleasure in daily living. This book reflects Dr. Manger's belief that a healthy adult life takes root in early childhood and is built on practices that are followed throughout life.

This volume adds a rich diversity of information that will help all of us not only in our own adult lives, but also in our work with the education and encouragement of young people. Dr. Manger has taken pains to delineate the priorities we must observe in planning our health routines, and he makes us intelligent participants in our attention to developing practices of sensible growth. This book takes us from the early years of childhood to all of the issues of adult living, and the reasons behind all of the doctor's advice are discussed in clear and helpful prose.

Dr. Manger has been working with schools to develop the use of a program he calls VITAL, an acronym for Values Initiative Teaching About Lifestyle. He emphasizes the importance of adult participation with children, whether in school or the home, and he always urges awareness of the necessity to develop strategies of prevention before damaging habits have taken hold in years of early adolescence.

If Americans can help growing youngsters develop self-confidence and commitment to healthy lifestyles, we will have given our youngsters the greatest possible tools of success and happiness. The first step on this road is a careful reading of Dr.

Manger's book and a willing participation in helping adults and children put all of this wonderful information into use.

Joan S. McMenamin
The Late Headmistress Emerita
The Nightingale-Bamford School
New York, NY

When I read the manuscript of *Our Greatest Threats*, I had an immediate reaction: "All Americans **should** read this. All people should be **required** to read this document before they are allowed to bring a new baby home from the maternity ward." It is hard to imagine a better gift for a new child than parents who know and practice the principles for healthy living presented here.

This is not a diet book. Oh, it is certainly true that those who follow Dr. Manger's advice will keep their weight under control. The book, however, is not about short-term weight loss, but about understanding and following principles that will lead to a healthy life, the sort of life we all want.

Why should every parent read it? Dr. Manger rightly points out that the habits of healthy living are best formed when one is young. Moreover, he knows what every good educator knows: example is the best way to influence a young person. That is why it is my fond hope, as an educator, that all parents will read this book and put it into practice in their lives and in the lives of their children. What a wonderful start for any child!

Moreover, I hope that those who are not the parents of young children will also read this book. It is a strange fact of human nature that when we are in good health we often take it for granted. However, when we are in ill health, we will do anything, give anything, to be restored. Dr. Manger shows us how to hold on to that treasure we know in our hearts is so important: good health.

This book performs three major tasks. First, it sets out the problems: what we are doing to ourselves as individuals and what we are doing to ourselves as a society. Second, it offers clear directions for how we should lead our lives to increase dramatically our chances to be healthy. It does not propose impossible goals demanding great self-sacrifice. It helps us to understand what simple steps will lead us to good health. Third, it gives us hope. Dr. Manger shows that **whenever** we start on the road to good health, positive results will occur. I was surprised to learn, for example, that the effects of tobacco smoking (even decades of it) can be reversed. This is a book that encourages and inspires.

We live in a time when we are all concerned about the threat of terrorist action against our people—and we are right to be concerned. However, what we are doing to ourselves is an even greater danger and is already causing the American people much greater damage. About 100,000 Americans die each year from complications related to obesity. The cost to the nation of diseases associated with obesity is about $117 billion a year. If any outside group or another nation caused 100,000 American deaths, our reaction would be extreme. Yet **each year** Americans do that to themselves. The book repeats the words of Dr. Jeffrey Koplan, former director of the Centers for Disease Control and Prevention, who began a lecture on bioterrorism with the statement that "the major threat to our nation is obesity and sedentary lifestyle."

This book is not just for the obese. All of those interested in health will find the pages on good nutrition a very helpful resource. Definitions, serving sizes, food groups, and the benefits and dangers of different foods are clearly spelled out. It is easy to introduce Dr. Manger's advice into one's daily living. He turns what could be a daunting challenge into a welcome opportunity.

This book, then, is for anyone who wants to lead the good life that can be enjoyed only when one has the blessing of health. The wise and detailed words of Dr. Manger set one on the path to attaining a most precious goal: good health. For your own sake, but even more for the sake of those who love you, *read this book.*

Mark H. Mullin
Headmaster Emeritus
Casady School, Oklahoma City, OK
Former Headmaster, St. Albans School, Washington, DC

I am an American who has always loved to travel. One disappointment I always feel, however, when I return to the country I love, is the realization that, in comparison to people of other countries, we are not a healthy people. For all of the money we spend on diet fads and personal trainers and yoga retreats, all too many of us are overweight, to cite only the most obvious example of our health risks, and at least by all appearances, year by year, we seem to be becoming even unhealthier.

I first met Bill Manger at a restaurant on the Lower East Side of Manhattan, near his office. The waiter knew Dr. Manger as a friend, but also as someone who was particular about what he ate and how he dressed for the weather and how, in fact, he lived his life. I know Dr. Manger as a great man. He is particular about his professional calling to medicine, his patriotic calling to citizenship, and his personal calling to his family and his friends and to the kind of life he believes we ought to live (in his presence I am often reminded of a Roman senator writing about life and the Republic). This latest book Dr. Manger has written captures his response to the concerns all of us share about our health in this country.

This book addresses all of the key aspects of good health—weight, exercise, salt, alcohol, smoking, drug use, sleep, sexually transmitted disease, and safety. It is an easy read in the best sense of the word "easy"—direct and plain spoken. There are lists, there are plans, and there are words of encouragement. It is—and this is why I hope for its success—an optimistic book. Dr. Manger, while being as current as any doctor on the best medical practices of the 21st century, still believes strongly in willpower. Here is the problem, the book says. Here is why the problem exists. Here is how best to achieve health. Now let's go forward.

I have been an educator for 30 years. I share Dr. Manger's passionate belief that education enlightens people to a better way of living. I urge you to acquaint yourself to the basic premises of this book and to share it and its educational plan with the people you know who work with children. As all of us know, habits are formed at a very early age. Although Dr. Manger is correct in saying that starting a healthy way of living at any age is effective for better health (consider the research on stopping smoking at any age), starting healthy habits as a child brings immeasurable benefits to one's life. I also believe, with Dr. Manger, that such individual benefits can only benefit the public. A less sedentary, healthy food-conscious, and mentally alert public makes for a more engaged citizenry.

I give my congratulations to Dr. Manger for his magnificent work.

Vance Wilson, Headmaster
St. Albans School
Washington, DC

As a headmaster who spent 30 years running two independent day schools in the Boston suburbs and in New York City, I have always been impressed by the way children absorb lessons in basic values from the age of 5 years, if not earlier. They are riveted in listening to presentations on safety issues and behavioral goals ("use your words, not your fists"). Just ask any 5- or 6-year old what he or she has learned in school about fire safety and/or being kind to others. They are also extremely interested in learning everything they can about taking care of animals, especially their domestic pets. In short, young children are completely open to lessons of *preventive* measures to control various aspects of their lives. Such knowledge gives them self-confidence and a sense of security, for what they fear most is that which they cannot control and that which they perceive their parents may be unable to control. More important, young children need to understand what they *can* control, for this empowers them to live without fear and to learn to appreciate the joys in life.

As children grow toward adolescence, a need beyond conquering fear and uncertainty develops, and that is the strength to withstand harmful peer pressure. Having the force of knowledge gives them the courage to resist temptations to join others in drug and alcohol abuse. It also gives them the power to control what their less secure friends and classmates may not, such as poor eating habits that could lead to eating disorders or obesity.

Whether it involves young children, adolescents, or adults, teaching does not always result in learning. The catalyst for learning is the application of what one has been taught, and the key to this is the belief that one has the ability and self-discipline to accomplish simple goals. In the school lives of young children the pattern of academic learning amounts basically to being shown a concept or process and then applying it with exercises and eventually being tested to determine quantitatively what has been learned. If children are given too much to absorb and lack confidence in what they have been taught, they will avoid the opportunity to apply what has been presented to them for fear of failure. A similar pattern develops with adults outside the controlled environment of classroom, only it is not just fear of failure that affects their level of application. Sometimes the perception is that the effort "isn't worth it" or that it "takes too much time." For example, it has been my experience that people with back problems will go to a doctor and receive a couple of pages of exercises to do and will follow them until their back no longer bothers them, yet physicians will frequently say that it is the exercise that one does when the back is not hurting that is likely to prevent further attacks. Why then do most back patients not continue the exercises? The answer is the lack of conviction that whatever time it takes is too much to spend on something that does not seem necessary. "If my back doesn't hurt, why should I do all of those exercises every day?"

For preventive care to work, the patient must believe that measures taken are doable. A set of exercises that takes 10 minutes a day are much more likely to be followed regularly than those that take 45 minutes. The prevalent concept that a daily half hour of walking can do a lot for heart health has many more people doing it who would never consider jogging or who felt incompetent to play tennis or skate. One other illustration of this point comes to mind. One day I was sitting in a faculty room when a young woman teacher on a diet, about to take a cookie from a tray on the coffee table asked, "What can you say to me that would stop me from doing this?" I said (without any qualifications in nutrition!), "It will add a half pound to your weight." Immediately, a big smile crossed her face as she put the cookie down, and she said, "I have to start thinking in those terms." She was given a preventive option that was both credible and easily accomplished because her motivation to control her weight *and* the simplicity of the act took precedence over her momentary temptation.

As a headmaster, I have always felt that general talks on the topic of safety in assemblies did more to make the speaker feel good than to curtail injuries among students. On the other hand, periodically offering specific steps students can take to avoid accidents or mishaps has a lasting effect, as I discovered in running a school in New York City. At least once a year we would have the local precinct of the N.Y.P.D. make a presentation to all of our students, and its list of "dos" and "don'ts" clearly stuck with the kids. This was impressively demonstrated whenever we quizzed them on various aspects of street safety. More important, we saw reassuring evidence of lessons learned whenever any of them actually faced dangerous situations on the streets. I have also observed that young children are more likely to put on their seat belts than many adults and that they frequently show concern for the smoking habits of adults in their lives. Someone has impressed them with the power of prevention!

When I first read this book, I felt it was clearly the most useful document I have ever come across on preventive measures for good health, for I found it to be extremely comprehensive yet very easy to read. The language is carefully selected to avoid medical terminology that could be meaningless to some or misunderstood by others. The graphics are superb, and the prescriptions for specific action are most helpful. For example, many health publications mention the dangers of smoking or the pitfalls of too much salt in the diet or the risks of alcohol abuse, yet do not offer explicit suggestions as to how these problems can be attacked successfully by the individual. In addition, what is offered here has the simplicity of application that will enable people to alter their habits by taking the responsibility to make the relatively minor changes that will improve their quality of life. In short, Dr. Manger makes a most convincing case that good health is mostly up to *you*.

Brian R. Walsh
Headmaster Emeritus
The Buckley School, New York City, NY
Former Headmaster
The Shore Country Day School
Beverly, MA

This is a delightful and informative book on the very timely subject of happy and healthy living. You don't "read" this book; it takes you on an easy journey into the world of looking better and feeling better. You will read about real people and how they discovered—or failed to discover—simple and fun ways to make their lives much better. There are many things that we can do to live the American Dream: to be an attractive, vibrant, and healthy person.

Take special note of "The Deadly Quartet" and blindness, the DASH diet of baskets of tasty food, more enjoyable smart sex without fear for infections and cancer, VITAL: one of the best kept secrets about teaching lifestyle to young people for a smart start to a lifetime of good living and success.

You will especially enjoy several personal stories—medical case studies of real people.

- "The Deadly Quartet," blindness, TV, and snacks
- Death of a President by a "silent killer"
- Booze, bleeding, and brain rot
- Doctors' doctors and diagnosis
- Smoking and slow death
- Sleeping
- Little known safety tips

The author is an experienced, compassionate, and seasoned physician, but more importantly, he loves life and people. He is an extraordinarily good communicator, as you will discover when you read this book.

With the girth of Americans expanding and all kinds of unhealthy temptations everywhere, our quality of life is declining along with our self-esteem. There is an increasing frequency of depression. Who better to sound the alarm and advise us about preventive and remedial action than a world-renowned internal medicine specialist? Dr. Manger projects enthusiasm and hope. *Our Greatest Threats* is admirably concise, clear, direct, and free of jargon. Because our memory is best served by repetition, the facts and advice are well-organized, but portions are repeated throughout the book. His advice, based on sound medical facts, is compelling. A special emphasis in this book is his concern about guiding young people to a healthy start in life. Young and old working together can help each other so very much!

You will keep the book in an accessible place so that you can use some parts as reference material. You will want to share the real-life stories with family and friends. With a little bit of encouragement, young people will use it like a special scouting guide. (Scouts take note for merit badges!) Not only can you improve yourself, but also you can give a good start to an entirely new generation by talking about the information in the book with young people.

The book is loaded with vital information. Our well-being depends on it. With great knowledge, wisdom, enthusiasm, and conviction, Dr. Manger informs, challenges, and inspires all those seeking healthier lives—young and old.

Ingrid Vaga Neel, MD
Assistant Professor of Pediatrics
Mayo Medical School
Rochester, MN
Certified by the Boards of Pediatrics and Adult and
Pediatric Allergy/Immunology

Honorable H. Bryan Neel, III, MD, PhD
Emeritus Professor and Past Chair
Department of Otolaryngology—Head and Neck Surgery
Mayo Clinic and Mayo Medical School
Rochester, MN
Regent Emeritus, University of Minnesota

Introduction

Good health is mostly up to *you*! This truth should be clear to all Americans. You must take it seriously, as **you and only you can change your lifestyle, your way of life.** Regrettably, in some parts of the world, many die from a lack of food, from malnutrition, and from various diseases because of inadequate prevention and lack of medicines, immunizations, vitamins, and sanitation. **Americans often die from the consequences of obesity from too much food, fat, and sugar, and from excess alcohol, excess salt, cigarette smoking, illicit drugs, some sexually transmitted diseases, and preventable injuries and diseases.** *You* are responsible for *your* lifestyle.

You *cannot* change your genes, age, sex, race, or family background, but you *can* avoid overeating. You *can* consume a healthy diet with less fat and sugar. You *can* get adequate exercise. You *can* limit the amount of dietary salt you eat. You *can* avoid drinking alcohol excessively. You *can* avoid cigarette smoking. You *can* avoid using marijuana or other illicit (street) drugs. You *can* avoid inadequate sleep. You *can* avoid acquiring sexually transmitted diseases, and you *can* observe safety precautions to help prevent injury and disease. **You *can*, therefore, change your lifestyle so that you can**

- Live safer
- Live healthier
- Live longer
- Feel better
- Look better
- Work better
- Play better
- Sleep better
- Improve your self-esteem
- Improve your quality of life
- Increase your energy
- Enjoy better sex

- Reduce stress
- Be happier

It is well established that your lifestyle can have an enormous impact on your health. **Everyone should know the major lifestyle risks: obesity, sedentary (physically inactive) lifestyle, excess salt and alcohol consumption, cigarette smoking, illicit drugs, and risky sexual activity.** Finally, because **injuries are the leading cause of death in individuals under 35 years of age,** this book also recommends ways of minimizing or avoiding serious injuries and fatalities. No matter your age, it is always essential to concentrate on changing an unhealthy lifestyle to a healthy lifestyle for the sake of your future health, self-esteem, and quality of life, as well as for the benefit of your family and associates.

Overeating—especially excess consumption of fat, sweets, snacks, and sugar—and drinking lots of sugar-laden sodas and other drinks and excess amounts of alcohol are major causes for the increase of obesity in the United States. Weight gain, then, may cause or aggravate hypertension (high blood pressure), adult-onset (type 2) diabetes, and osteoarthritis, and it may elevate cholesterol and other harmful fats in the blood. Obesity may also cause sleep apnea (when breathing stops periodically during sleep). This can result in severe elevations of blood pressure, heart irregularities, and occasionally death. Some of these consequences of obesity are being detected in children in greater numbers than ever before. It is evident that overweight and obesity in children can impair self-esteem, performance in schoolwork, athletic ability, and quality of life, and it can cause despair and depression. We are correctly warned that our **children are growing up in a toxic food and beverage environment.**

Unfortunately, we are constantly bombarded by advertisements for food, snacks, and drinks that encourage us to eat and drink more.

The abundance of food and non-nutritious drinks and the erosion of exercise time by television, computers, and the availability of convenient transportation provide an environment that contributes to the crisis of obesity in our nation.

In addition to the ill effects of overeating, there are other types of serious but relatively rare eating disorders such as anorexia nervosa and bulimia. About 90% of these conditions occur in white girls and young women and are associated with extreme psychologic disturbances. Anorexia nervosa can cause extreme undernutrition, malnutrition, weight loss, debilitation, and sometimes death. Individuals with bulimia are frequent binge eaters who periodically gorge themselves with food and then discharge the food through self-induced vomiting and the excessive use of laxatives. Individuals with either of these conditions are very fearful of gaining weight and becoming obese. Marked weight loss occurs in anorexia nervosa but usually is not pronounced in individuals with bulimia. To avoid obesity and maintain a normal weight, "healthy nutrition" rather than "dieting" should be emphasized, as dieting is occasionally the gateway to bulimia and anorexia. In this book, however, we will focus only on obesity as an eating disorder, one of our greatest health threats.

Excessive salt consumption also can aggravate or cause hypertension in individuals who are sensitive to salt. Hypertension, diabetes, and elevated harmful blood fats result in hardening of the arteries, which can impair the blood supply to various parts of the body and lead to heart and kidney damage and failure, stroke, and poor circulation in the legs. Furthermore, a high-fat diet has been linked to some cancers—especially colon cancer.

Cigarette smoking is largely responsible for lung cancer and also serious breathing problems, such as emphysema, which impairs the ability of the lungs to take in enough oxygen for the blood. Excess alcohol consumption adds more calories and increases weight with no nutritional benefit. Excess alcohol also can cause hypertension, and chronic alcoholism can damage the liver, brain, heart, and nerves. Complications of arterial disease, especially damage of the arteries to the heart, brain, and kidneys, account for 50% of all deaths in the United States each year; cancer causes about 22% of deaths.

There is no excuse for not trying to protect your health and the health of your family. What could be more important?

The purpose of this book is to present facts that will encourage you to take the necessary steps to change or, at least, improve your lifestyle and benefit your health and that of your family. However, *motivation* **(a strong desire) is absolutely essential for success in achieving and maintaining a healthy lifestyle.** Information and education about the serious hazards of an unhealthy lifestyle and urging individuals to change and improve their lifestyle and health may be helpful; however, again, **motivation is the key to success, and that depends on you! The greatest enemy of motivation is "fear of failure."**

It is frequently said that "knowledge is power," yet success in almost any endeavor depends not only on knowledge but also on commitment and perseverance. If you will accept these truths, you can achieve better health and greater happiness for you and your family.

A major aim of this book is to inform you that a healthy diet and moderate, regular exercise play an extremely important role in protecting your health. A healthy diet can maintain a reasonably normal weight, vital to preventing or minimizing some of the most common serious diseases in Americans, namely, hypertension, hardening of the arteries, heart and kidney disease, stroke, diabetes, and some types of cancer. The magnitude of the problems of obesity, lack of exercise, hypertension, and their complications is discussed. The role of salt or alcohol in the cause or aggravation of hypertension is considered. **Then a very simple dietary approach will be presented—one that** *definitely* **can reduce weight if necessary, lower or prevent elevated blood pressure, reduce the chance of stroke, reduce elevated fats in the blood, and even improve or prevent diabetes.** Because of the extraordinarily damaging effects of cigarette smoking, this book also considers this serious health hazard and recommends ways to deal with this deadly problem. Finally, the serious consequences of smoking marijuana, using other illicit drugs, and engaging in risky sex behavior are addressed briefly.

Effective prevention is always far better than treating a disease. It therefore seems especially important for schools to provide the proper guidance and opportunity for good nutrition and exercise at a very young age—to preschool and kindergarten children, and first and second graders—when they are particularly receptive and eager to learn. The importance of healthy nutrition and adequate exercise should be repeated and reinforced as the child grows older. At appropriate ages, education about the risks of cigarette smoking, the use of illicit drugs or alcohol, and sexual activities and ways of minimizing injuries should be introduced and discussed repeatedly at all subsequent grade levels until high school graduation. Parents have an obligation to participate in this vital educational process. The future lives of many children will benefit greatly by early education and implementation of healthy lifestyles. **Establishing healthy lifestyles early affords the greatest opportunity for good health throughout your life.**

A program entitled VITAL (Values Initiative Teaching About Lifestyle) has been developed and introduced to some preschool, kindergarten, and first and second grade children. The enthusiasm for this program shown by children, teachers, educational professionals, pediatricians, and parents has been extremely positive and gratifying. However, measuring the success of the program necessarily will require some years of experience with it and observations of its beneficial effects.

This book is written, with the help of many outstanding consultants with a wide range of expertise, to improve the health of our nation by establishing beneficial lifestyles.

Overweight and Obesity Crisis

Americans face a most serious health crisis, namely, obesity, which can cause hypertension, type 2 adult-onset diabetes, elevated harmful blood fats, and many cancers. These complications are responsible for over 100,000 deaths each year! The annual cost of diseases attributable to obesity is reported to be $117 billion. As aptly stated in a recent editorial, "Fat is a fiscal issue." The word *crisis* is composed of two characters in the Chinese language: *danger* and *opportunity*. This definition of crisis seems eminently fitting and appealing because it suggests a possible turning point for "better or worse"; it implies that we have the "opportunity" to correct unhealthy lifestyles and protect our future well-being and the health of our children.

Dr. Jeffrey Koplan, former Director of the Centers for Disease Control and Prevention, began a lecture on bioterrorism with the statement that **the major threat to our nation is obesity and sedentary lifestyle.** What a powerful and thought-provoking statement!

As Dr. Stephen Bloom of the Imperial College Faculty of Medicine in London says, "We've got a major epidemic sweeping the world, causing a massive increase in death." Dr. George Yancopoulos, Chief Scientific Officer and President of Regeneron Laboratories in Tarrytown, New York, further states that "obesity is the most dangerous epidemic facing mankind, and we are relatively unprepared for it." Drs. Jack and Susan Vanovski of the National Institutes of Health point out that "one of the most compelling challenges of the 21st century is to develop effective strategies to prevent and treat pediatric obesity."

Dr. Jeffrey Friedman, a leading obesity researcher at Rockefeller University and discoverer of leptin (a weight-regulating hormone) further states, "Food consumes our interest. To the hungry, it is the focal point of every thought and action. To the hundreds of millions of obese and overweight individuals, it is the siren's song, a constant temptation that must be avoided lest one suffer health consequences and stigmatization. To the non-obese, it is a source of sustenance and often pleasure. To the food and diet industries, it is big business. And to those interested in public health, it is at the root of one of the most pressing public health problems in the developed and developing world" (*Science*, February 7, 2003).

Genetic, hormonal, and environmental factors appear to be involved in the development of obesity; however, currently, to combat obesity, we must depend on controlling the amount of food calories we consume and the amount of calories we burn by physical activity. More research is needed to develop new drugs that are effective in causing weight loss.

Sadly, excess weight and obesity (which means that because of fat accumulation your weight is at least 20% above what you should weigh) are rampant throughout the United States. It is reported that since 1960 the average weight of adult Americans has increased about 25 pounds, and the average dress size for women has increased from 8 to 14. Currently, there are about 60 million obese adult Americans. **Unfortunately, the culture and environment in the United States encourage overeating and a sedentary lifestyle.** Obesity not only is of epidemic proportions in this country, but also is increasing rapidly in most of the world. In 1988, the then Surgeon General, Dr. C. Everett Koop, correctly warned Americans that "one personal choice seems to influence long-term health more than any other: *what we eat.*"

A simple way to determine your approximate ideal weight is the following:

- For men, use 106 pounds for the first 5 feet and then add 6 pounds for each additional inch of height.
- For women, use 100 pounds for the first 5 feet and then add 5 pounds for each additional inch of height.

You can also determine your approximate ideal weight from Table 1.

Table 1	Height and Weight Standards

These are 1983 Metropolitan Life tables showing desirable weight related to size of frame (body build), for those 25 to 59 years old, in shoes with 1-inch heels and wearing 5 pounds of clothing for men and 3 pounds of clothing for women.

Men				Women			
Height	Small	Medium	Large	Height	Small	Medium	Large
5' 2"	128–134	131–141	138–150	4' 10"	102–111	109–121	118–131
5' 3"	130–136	133–143	140–153	4' 11"	103–113	111–123	120–134
5' 4"	132–138	135–145	142–156	5' 0"	104–115	113–126	122–137
5' 5"	134–140	137–148	144–160	5' 1"	106–118	115–129	125–140
5' 6"	136–142	139–151	146–164	5' 2"	108–121	118–132	128–143
5' 7"	138–145	142–154	149–168	5' 3"	111–124	121–135	131–147
5' 8"	140–148	145–157	152–172	5' 4"	114–127	124–138	134–151
5' 9"	142–151	148–160	155–176	5' 5"	117–130	127–141	137–155
5' 10"	144–154	151–163	158–180	5' 6"	120–133	130–144	140–159
5' 11"	146–157	154–166	161–184	5' 7"	123–136	133–147	143–163
6' 0"	149–160	157–170	164–188	5' 8"	126–139	136–150	146–167
6' 1"	152–164	160–174	168–192	5' 9"	129–142	139–153	149–170
6' 2"	155–168	164–178	172–197	5' 10"	132–145	142–156	152–173
6' 3"	158–172	167–182	176–202	5' 11"	135–148	145–159	155–176
6' 4"	162–176	171–187	181–207	6' 0"	138–151	148–16	158–179

However, estimates of body weight (even standard height–weight tables) do not indicate whether you are fat.

A more accurate way to determine whether your weight is excessive and might contribute to health problems is to determine your body mass index (BMI). For most individuals, BMI correlates with total body fat and with risk for health problems (Table 2). BMI can be determined by dividing your weight in kilograms by the square of your height in meters (kg/m^2). If you prefer to use pounds and inches to determine BMI, divide the weight in pounds by the square of your height in inches and then multiplying by 703. For example, if you weigh 160 pounds and are 70 inches tall, then

$$\left(\frac{160}{70 \times 70}\right) \times 703 = \left(\frac{160}{4,900}\right) \times 703 = \text{a BMI of about } 22.9$$

You can also use the BMI calculator at www.nhlbisupport.com/bmi. A BMI index of 19 to 24 is considered desirable, 25 to 29 overweight, 30 or over obesity, and 40 or over termed *morbid obesity*, as it is such a serious health hazard. Table 2 can help you determine whether you are overweight or obese.

Table 2	BMI											
	Healthy		Overweight					Obesity				
BMI	19	24	25	26	27	28	29	30	35	40	45	50
Height							Weight in Pounds					
4' 10"	91	115	119	124	129	134	138	143	167	191	215	239
4' 11"	94	119	124	128	133	138	143	148	173	198	222	247
5' 0"	97	123	128	133	138	143	148	153	179	204	230	255
5' 1"	100	127	132	137	143	148	153	158	185	211	238	264
5' 2"	104	131	136	142	147	153	158	164	191	218	246	273
5' 3"	107	135	141	146	152	158	163	169	197	225	254	282
5' 4"	110	140	145	151	157	163	169	174	204	232	262	291
5' 5"	114	144	150	156	162	168	174	180	210	240	270	300
5' 6"	118	148	155	161	167	173	179	186	216	247	278	309
5' 7"	121	153	159	166	172	178	185	191	223	255	287	319
5' 8"	125	158	164	171	177	184	190	197	230	262	295	328
5' 9"	128	162	169	176	182	189	196	203	236	270	304	338
5' 10"	132	167	174	181	188	195	202	209	243	278	313	348
5' 11"	136	172	179	186	193	200	208	215	250	286	322	358
6' 0"	140	177	184	191	199	206	213	221	258	294	331	368
6' 1"	144	182	189	197	204	212	219	227	265	302	340	378
6' 2"	148	186	194	202	210	218	225	233	272	311	350	389
6' 3"	152	192	200	208	216	224	232	240	279	319	359	399
6' 4"	156	197	205	213	221	230	238	246	287	328	369	410

Modified from National Institutes of Health. Clinical guidelines on the identification, evaluation and treatment of overweight and obesity in adults. *Mayo Clinic on High Blood Pressure* 1998.

Determination of BMI in children requires the interpretation by a physician because it depends not only on weight and height but also on gender and age. However, parents should become concerned that their child is significantly overweight if the child develops abdominal obesity and requires oversized clothes compared with children of the same age.

We are the fattest nation in the world! A national health and nutrition survey by the government in 2002 revealed that 65% of adult Americans were overweight, and 31% were obese. (Obesity in the United Kingdom [22%], Germany [11.5%], France [9%], and Japan [3.2%] was significantly less.) In the United States, 34% of women and 28% of men are obese; 5% of Americans are morbidly or superobese, and obesity is more prevalent in Americans with low income. This increase in the prevalence of obesity has been called "The Larding of America." The number of obese adults has doubled in the past 20 years, and there is a pronounced weight gain with aging, as individuals become less active and have less muscle to burn up calories. In addition, the number of overweight and obese children and adolescents in the United States has almost tripled since 1980. More than 10% of children 2 through 5 years old, about 15% of children between 6 and 11 years old, and 15% of teenagers are overweight, and almost 13% of children are obese. In the past decade, type 2 diabetes has increased 10-fold in children. It is now estimated that one in eight children will develop type 2 diabetes! If this increased trend toward obesity continues, life expectancy in this nation may indeed begin to decrease in the near future by 2 to 5 years! A recent school program in Boston sends home health report cards with information about student weight and physical fitness in an effort to get the attention of parents and their help in combating childhood obesity.

It is particularly disturbing that some turnstiles at Disney World and some bus seats have been enlarged to accommodate obese individuals. Equally disturbing is the marked increased demand for large coffins (44 inches across compared with 24 inches for standard caskets), increased burial plot size (from 3 to 4 feet wide), and for larger hearses. Most crematoria cannot cremate bodies over 500 pounds, and there is now a surcharge on embalming and transporting very obese individuals.

In her book, *Food Politics*, Dr. Marion Nestle, professor and former chair of the Department of Nutrition and Food Studies at New York University, depicts how the food industry has succeeded in manipulating Americans to consume more food and beverages. Much of the marketing has focused on foods that are high in fat and sugar and on soft drinks; the consumption of these drinks has more than doubled since 1970. The food industry spends about $33 billion yearly marketing food, some of which is highly caloric and low in nutrition ("junk food"), to promote greater sales and consumption. Sadly, the success of this relentless food promotion is closely correlated with increased obesity in the United States. Recently, food companies have targeted a particularly vulnerable group—children and members of minority groups. The result has been a progressive increase in caloric consumption and progressive fattening of America. Excessive weight and obesity, coupled with a sedentary lifestyle, are seriously impairing the health of our nation and significantly adding to the skyrocketing cost of health care. The sensible dictum "eat less and move more" has been relatively ineffective, practiced by only a small percentage of the public. It is reported that children spend more time watching TV than in any other activity and that they are exposed to 20,000 commercials (about 150 to 200 hours) yearly. Unfortunately, most advertisements do not encourage a healthy diet and practically never promote consumption of fruits and vegetables.

There is growing anger by **some of the public who claim that certain fast-food restaurants are responsible for their obesity and obesity of their children. This claim denies personal responsibility for**

their eating habits and appears an unjustified accusation with little merit. The fast-food industry and restaurants could help alleviate the problem by offering some guidance and information regarding calories, fat, and sugar content of their food and drinks.

Most public schools offer students lunches (paid for by the government) that contain reasonable nutrition. However, 20% of schools also sell pizzas, burgers, and fries from some of the fast-food restaurants, and many schools have vending machines that dispense food, snacks, and soft drinks that are often loaded with fat and sugar. No school should have to depend on funds from restaurant chains that dictate the type of foods and drinks that are available to their students and staff. The unfortunate consequence is that most children and teenagers consume some food and drinks high in calories that result in weight gain and obesity. It has been suggested that soda substitutes include bottled water, 100% fruit juice, and milk. Dr. Koplan warns that the nation's health is threatened through poor eating and drinking habits and a lack of physical activity. As a nation, we literally are on a collision course to greater disease, disability, and death from lifestyle factors that we can control. Fortunately, concern about marketing these foods and drinks to children has increased, and vending machines have been removed from the premises of some schools.

Food or a lack of food causes substances to be released from the stomach, intestine, and fat cells that signal the brain and thereby cause a person to eat or to stop eating. **Although a genetic abnormality may account for some imbalance in these signals that could result in overeating, it appears that environmental factors—especially excess consumption of fat and products containing sugar and physical inactivity—play the major role in weight gain and obesity.** It has been said that "genes may load the gun, but environment pulls the trigger." Because we cannot alter our genes, we must change our lifestyle to a program of healthy nutrition and physical activity. The fact that body metabolism (the ability of the body to metabolize or burn up food) decreases with aging and individuals usually become less active as they grow older partly explains an increase in body weight without any change in food or calorie consumption. Of paramount importance is that we recognize the seriousness of obesity and the many diseases and problems with which it is associated. **Your chance of developing hypertension if you are obese may be eight times greater than that of normal-weight individuals. Hypertension occurs in approximately 50% of obese individuals.** Obesity is the most important lifestyle factor causing or aggravating hypertension. It predisposes a person to or aggravates cardiovascular disease (hardening of the arteries, heart failure, and stroke). The occurrence of obesity at a young age may lead to the early development of heart and blood vessel disease and other complications. About 3% of children in the United States have hypertension, which is often the result of obesity; another 10% are considered at risk for developing hypertension.

The consequences of obesity are numerous, such as impaired action of insulin and increased glucose (sugar), cholesterol, and other unhealthy fats in the blood. These lead to the development of adult-onset (type 2) diabetes and hardening of the arteries. It is estimated that 20 million Americans have diabetes, and an additional 40 to 60 million have a tendency to develop diabetes. About 95% of these diabetics are obese. **Adult-onset diabetes is extremely rare in persons with a BMI below 22 (for normal weight, see Table 2), indicating that this type of diabetes may usually be prevented by maintaining a normal weight,** even in individuals who have a genetic predisposition to develop this disease. Recently, it has been reported that overweight and obesity may also hasten the onset of type 1 diabetes, which occurs in children and young adults. Ninety percent of diabetics have type 2 diabetes, which results from an inability of adequate or excess amounts of insulin to metabolize food normally. Type 1 diabetes results from the pancreas's inadequate production of insulin.

Reduced lung capacity with impaired breathing, sleep apnea, gall-stones, degenerative osteoarthritis (sometimes causing severe disability), varicose veins and blood clots, and hypertension in pregnancy may also be consequences of obesity. Recently, it has been established that increased body weight is associated with higher death rates in men and women from cancers of the esophagus (swallowing tube), colon, rectum, liver, gall bladder, pancreas, kidney, and some malignancies involving the lymph tissue and bone marrow. Increased weight is also associated with higher death rates from stomach and prostate cancer in men and from cancers of the uterus, cervix, ovary, and breast in women. It is estimated that overweight and obesity could account for 14% of all cancer deaths in men and 20% in women.

Obesity makes surgery more difficult. Wounds do not heal as fast, and infections are more common. All such medical problems can increase your doctor, medicine, and hospital bills. The considerably lower prevalence of obesity in older persons is explained by the fact that most people who are significantly overweight die at a younger age than persons of normal weight.

It has been reported that obesity is more strongly linked with chronic diseases than with living in poverty, cigarette smoking, or alcohol consumption. Medical consequences and complications are not only enormous for the obese population, but the healthcare costs of these complications affect everyone.

Let us first examine the serious health risks associated with overweight and especially obesity.

Figure 1 indicates the complications often related to obesity. **More than 100,000 Americans die each year from some of these complications, and the cost of diseases associated with overweight and obesity is about $117 billion a year, half of which is paid by the government.**

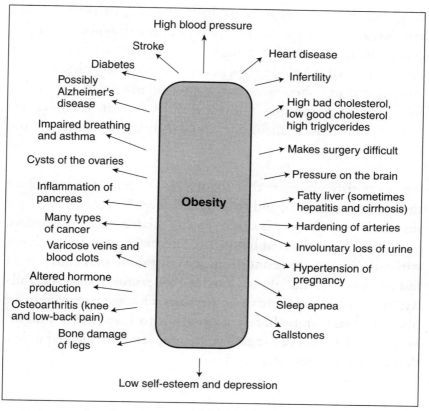

Figure 1 Conditions that might occur with obesity.

Figures 2–4 indicate the consequences of some of these complications. **The combination of abdominal obesity, high blood pressure, diabetes or elevated blood sugar, elevated triglycerides (harmful blood fats), and decreased protective high-density lipoprotein (HDL) cholesterol, is known as the metabolic syndrome and had been given the title of "The Deadly Quartet"!** However, the condition exists if an individual has any three to five of these risk factors. In addition, individuals with this syndrome tend to have high levels of C-reactive protein (CRP) in their blood, which is an indication of inflammation that may cause heart disease. The metabolic syndrome seems to be a major contributor to heart disease, stroke, hardening of the arteries, and kidney damage, even though individuals with this condition may not have a high level of harmful low-density lipoprotein (LDL) cholesterol in their blood. Hispanics, African Americans, and obese persons are particularly prone to develop this harmful syndrome. The good news is that losing excess weight may reduce all of the abnormalities occurring in the metabolic syndrome.

Recent statistics indicate that about 25% of adult Americans have this serious syndrome, and roughly 50% over 50 years of age have the syndrome! Obesity is often directly related to the occurrence of hypertension, elevated blood fats, and diabetes in adults. **Even without these related conditions, obesity alone may cause heart failure. The fact that obesity can lead to serious disease, disability, or death should convince persons who are overweight or obese to start immediately a program to lose excess weight.** However, despite a desire to lose weight, very few succeed unless they are firmly committed to do so.

Case Report

R.N. is an African American who recalls being obese when he was only 12 years old. At that time, he was about 5 feet tall and weighed 195 pounds. A physical education program was not required in his school, and he rarely exercised; sports were not enjoyable because his weight markedly limited his ability to run and participate effectively as a team player. As a result, he usually spent 6 to 7 hours daily watching television from a couch, while constantly eating high-calorie snacks and drinking large amounts of sugar-laden sodas. Most of his meals consisted of fast foods with a high concentration of fat, few fruits and vegetables, and lots of sodas and ice cream. He also says that he always liked to add salt to his food.

R.N. did not finish high school, and he continued to overeat and avoid any exercise except walking when necessary. By the time he was 30 years old, he weighed 285 pounds and was 5 feet 6 inches tall. His blood pressure was found to be very high (210/120), and it was discovered that he had type 2 diabetes and a very high level of harmful fats in his blood. This combination (abdominal obesity, diabetes, elevated blood fats, and hypertension)—"The Deadly Quartet"—indicates a very high risk for cardiovascular disease. It was particularly important that he seek medical treatment promptly and change to a healthier lifestyle.

Unfortunately, he delayed treatment until his eyesight became impaired as a result of hemorrhages and damage of the blood vessels in the back of his eyes—the consequence of hypertension and diabetes. He also experienced shortness of breath with even mild exertion, which resulted from enlargement of his heart and heart failure. He then sought medical treatment, but his blood pressure and diabetes were poorly controlled. When only 35 years old, he suffered a massive stroke, which resulted in severe weakness of his right arm and leg, accompanied by impairment of his ability to talk distinctly.

Sadly, his physical limitations prevent his working and supporting his wife and two young children. If R.N. had only maintained a normal weight, he probably would not have developed diabetes and the marked elevation of fats in his blood. He also may not have developed severe hypertension, although excess use of salt may increase blood pressure over time, particularly in salt-sensitive African Americans. Today, his diabetes, blood pressure, and blood fats are under good control, but the damage has been done.

Hypertension is an enormous health problem in the United States and in the rest of the world. It afflicts more than 65 million adult Americans, and it is more common, more severe, and more

deadly in African Americans. About 30% of hypertensive individuals do not know that their blood pressure is elevated, and only 34% have their pressure properly controlled. Hypertension can damage arteries throughout the body, and these arteries can become partly or completely blocked and impair blood flow—especially in the heart, brain, kidneys, eyes, and legs. As a result, hypertension is a major cause of strokes, heart attacks, heart and kidney failure, poor circulation in the legs, and visual impairment. Hypertension may be responsible for 75% of strokes and 90% of heart failure cases. It is the major contributor to 1 million deaths and 1 million disabilities each year.

The good news is that with appropriate medication and lifestyle changes, complications from hypertension can be prevented or minimized. Previous to the development of effective antihypertensive medication, little could be done to prevent these complications.

Case Report

F.D.R. was found to have an elevated blood pressure of 170/90 when he was 57 years old (normal blood pressure is less than 140/90). He was not overweight; however, his ability to exercise was limited because his legs were paralyzed from polio. He was advised to rest and was given medication to help him relax. Antihypertensive medication was not yet available to lower blood pressure. Over the next 6 years, F.D.R.'s blood pressure continued to increase and often reached levels of 220/120. By then, he had symptoms of heart failure, and his kidneys began to fail. At this point, little could be done to prevent further complications. In 1945, while he was on a brief vacation, he suffered a massive brain hemorrhage. This ended the life of President Franklin Delano Roosevelt at the young age of 63.

Almost certainly, if President Roosevelt had been treated with some of the antihypertensive drugs now available when his hypertension was first detected, he would not have suffered a massive stroke and might have lived many more years. His untimely death emphasizes the importance of early recognition and treatment of this "silent killer," hypertension.

The main concern about overweight and obesity, of course, should be health and not appearance; however, obesity can have an im-

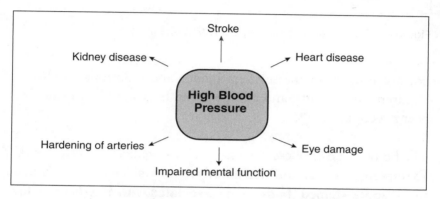

Figure 2 Conditions that might occur with high blood pressure.

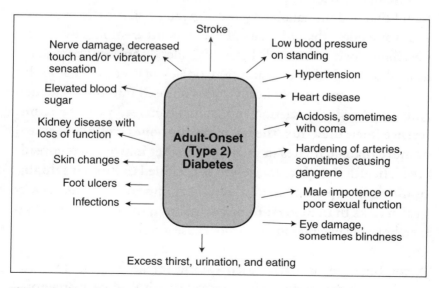

Figure 3 Conditions that might occur with adult-onset diabetes.

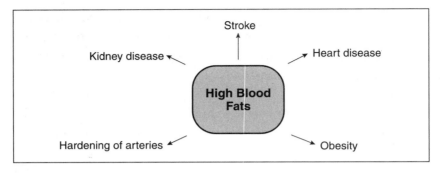

Figure 4 Conditions that might occur with high blood fats.

portant impact on the self-confidence and emotional health of children, adolescents, and adults. It can be a significant cause of peer rejection.

The body shape of obese persons can be a predictor of health risk. **Extra weight that is confined mainly to the waist has been likened to an "apple-shaped" body and is associated with a higher risk for heart disease, hypertension, stroke, elevated blood cholesterol, and diabetes.** Researchers at Columbia Medical Center recently found that abdominal obesity was a greater risk for stroke in men and women less than 65 years of age than other stroke risk factors (i.e., high blood pressure, diabetes, high blood cholesterol, smoking, heart disease, alcohol consumption, or lack of exercise). Fat in this area is very active metabolically and is released into the circulation and can cause inflammation and arterial damage. **A waist circumference (measured from the top of the hip bones around the waist) of more than 40 inches in men or 35 inches in women is considered a health risk. If extra weight is confined to hips and thighs, resulting in a "pear-shaped" body, there appears to be no greater health risks than in persons of normal weight.** Fat in this area is metabolically inactive and does not cause arterial damage.

A combination of a decreased caloric intake and an increased caloric expenditure through increased physical activity or aerobic exercise is essential for successful weight reduction. However, **the key ingredient for losing weight and maintaining weight reduction is *motivation* and *commitment*.** For various medical reasons, some individuals may be unable to increase their physical activity; however, everyone has the ability to curtail overeating and combat this "hand-to-mouth" disease. Orson Welles, the late movie star, confessed, "My doctor told me to stop having intimate dinners for four unless there are three other people." Unfortunately, he did not follow his doctor's advice.

Changing from an unhealthy to a healthy lifestyle may not only save your life, but also may have an enormous beneficial impact on your family, particularly your children. What could be more important than the health of your children? Albert Schweitzer, the great humanitarian, said that "example is not the most important thing in influencing others, it is the *only* thing." Parents should be good role models by healthful eating and engaging in regular physical activity, together with their children whenever possible. Parental participation in helping their children discover a healthy lifestyle is extremely valuable. Your actions and lifestyle can strongly influence those around you, especially young children. A noteworthy medical report in the *Archives of Family Medicine* revealed that children who dined with their family, if their family ate a healthful dinner, were more likely to eat nutritious food than when they are on their own. Parents' good example influenced children to eat more vegetables and fruits, to drink more milk and less sodas, and to eat less fried, high-fat, and sugary foods. **Improving your health should be a basic desire; however, benefiting the health of your children is an *obligation*!**

The problem with most books that deal with diet is that food portions, weights, and caloric value of foods are not presented in a way that can be easily understood and used. As a consequence, many readers become confused and unwilling to spend the effort and time to prepare a diet schedule that will reduce their weight, lessen their hypertension, decrease elevated blood fats, and improve their diabetes. Some may lose interest and make no attempt to improve their lifestyle unless the diet is easy to prepare and follow.

It is most desirable to select a healthy diet that has been approved by the medical profession. This diet also should be helpful in preventing and controlling weight, blood pressure, blood cholesterol, and diabetes. The diet should not require any special understanding of nutrition. The food should be simple to prepare and delicious. You should learn to read food and beverage labels to improve your knowledge of the fat, sugar, salt content, and caloric values of foods.

Moderation in everything we do is central to our well-being and health. Eating excess amounts of high-caloric foods can be just as dangerous to your health as drinking excess alcohol or smoking. Overeating in general, especially of high-calorie, high-fat foods and drinks in combination with a sedentary lifestyle, will result in excess body fat accumulation and weight gain. The United States now has an epidemic of obesity. In recognition of the seriousness of this epidemic, recently, the **Internal Revenue Service has designated obesity a serious disease and permits tax deductions of certain weight-loss programs as a medical expense.**

An unhealthy diet high in calories coupled with a lack of physical activity is the major cause of weight gain and obesity. Genetic abnormalities may drive some to eat more and yet not experience the normal sensation of being full after a meal. However, this should not interfere with your ability to lose weight if you are willing and committed to reduce your consumption of food calories and if you will increase the calories you burn with daily physical activity.

Many Americans are "hooked" on food prepared by the $129 billion fast-food industry, which is constantly expanding throughout the nation. It is estimated that more than half of the money spent on fast food comes from drive-thru lanes. That is why so many fast-food restaurants are adding "drive-thru" facilities and constantly are seeking ways to deliver food faster. Many people, unwilling to be inconvenienced or to expend the energy to get out of their car, demand fast service.

Often, restaurant meals contain more fat, cholesterol, and salt than home-cooked meals and are lower in calcium, potassium, and fiber. **The average adult American does not need more than 2,000 to 2,800 calories in the daily diet unless he or she is very active. Unfortunately, many meals served in restaurants may contain 1,500–2,000 calories for a *single* meal.** Even some dinner plates have increased in size from 10.5 to 12.5 inches.

Of great concern is the trend to offer larger amounts of food and sodas ("super-sized" portions) at many fast-food restaurants. For example, in the mid-1950s, the combination of a hamburger, cola, and fries amounted to about 590 calories; today, a quarter-pound cheeseburger, super-sized fries, and super-sized cola are equivalent to 1,550 calories! A double hamburger with cheese, super-sized fries, and super-sized cola add up to 2,050 calories—almost as many calories as the average adult should consume in 1 day! The enormous growth since 1955 of serving sizes of three popular products is graphically illustrated in **Figure 5.**

The fast-food industry continues to offer super-sized portions. Additional concerns are that fast foods are becoming more available in schools in the United States and that about 50% of school districts have signed contracts with soft-drink makers. Efforts are being made by some of the fast-food chains (e.g., McDonald's, Burger King, Subway, Pizza Hut, Taco Bell, Hardees, and KFC) to offer choices of healthier food and smaller portions with fewer calories. However, most of the public seems unwilling to change dietary habits significantly. Indeed, much more must be done to educate the public, particularly young children, to make the

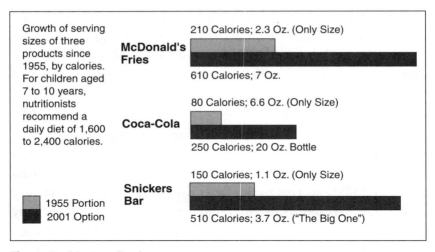

Growth of serving sizes of three products since 1955, by calories. For children aged 7 to 10 years, nutritionists recommend a daily diet of 1,600 to 2,400 calories.

McDonald's Fries
210 Calories; 2.3 Oz. (Only Size)
610 Calories; 7 Oz.

Coca-Cola
80 Calories; 6.6 Oz. (Only Size)
250 Calories; 20 Oz. Bottle

1955 Portion
2001 Option

Snickers Bar
150 Calories; 1.1 Oz. (Only Size)
510 Calories; 3.7 Oz. ("The Big One")

Figure 5   Monster Portions
Source: Center for Science in the Public Interest.

proper choices and to follow a healthier diet. For example, most parents are unaware that chicken nuggets sold by fast-food chains contain about 57% fat calories (almost twice the amount in an ordinary hamburger). Many young children regularly eat chicken nuggets, and this may result in a preference for fatty foods as they grow older. Chicken nuggets, currently a very popular food item for both children and adults, can and should be prepared so that they contain mainly chicken and some carbohydrate but very little fat.

Most do not appreciate that just a 12-ounce container of a sugar-sweetened carbonated soda contains 39 grams of sugar (about 9.5 teaspoonfuls). Soft drinks have very little nutritional value, and they have been called "liquid candy." Only diet sodas have no sugar added; instead, they contain a harmless noncaloric sweetener. Also, most iced tea, lemonade, and many fruit drinks similarly have very high sugar content, and their use should be limited; instead, water or low-caloric or diet drinks should be consumed more frequently. It is recommended that diet colas be decaffeinated, as excess consumption of caffeine can cause insomnia, nervousness, irritability, difficulty in relaxing, anxiety, shakiness, and panic attacks. It can also temporarily increase the heart rate and cause heart irregularities.

Black tea and green tea contain only one half to one fourth of the amount of caffeine present in an 8-ounce cup of coffee. Tea is a good source of antioxidants, which appear protective against a number of diseases. Furthermore, regular consumption of tea may be associated with higher bone density. (Herbal teas are not really teas but rather a combination of herbs, fruits, and spices.)

Some summer coffee drinks also contain coconut, chocolate, whipped cream, brownie pieces, and mocha syrup and, therefore, of course, a heavy load of calories. **Consumption of alcohol also adds extra calories with no nutritional value.** It should not be surprising that unwise beverage choices can add calories and increase weight. However, there is evidence that a modest amount of alcohol may be beneficial to some adults, especially those with coronary heart disease.

Is there any wonder that weight gain is inevitable, as so many Americans consume so many more calories than they should? It also is unfortunate that, as children, many of us were told to eat every bit of food on our plates. **Some adults probably are conditioned to feel that eating everything on their plates is almost a duty.** However, some restaurants permit ordering just half a portion of a food item. Ordering smaller portions or sharing full portions with a spouse or friend will save money and benefit your health by avoiding excess calories.

It is well to recall that we should "eat to live—not live to eat!" When Mae West, the late movie actress, said that too much of a good thing can be wonderful, we who remember her films know that she was not talking about food.

Overweight and Obesity Crisis

Many Americans eat far too much fat, often up to 40% of the calories in their diet; the dietary Guidelines for Americans recommend no more than 30% of the calories, with only 10% from saturated fat and the rest from monounsaturated or polyunsaturated fat. Some very healthy fats are present in olive, canola, sunflower, and safflower oils; fish oils; avocados; and nuts. However, there is some evidence that when these oils are used to fry foods, a toxic compound is produced that may be harmful to your health. Sources of unhealthy fats are animal fats, dairy products, nondairy creamers, shortening, some margarines, and palm and coconut oils. Every gram of fat has 9 calories, whereas every gram of carbohydrate or protein contains only 4 calories. Therefore, the same amount of fat supplies more than twice as many calories as carbohydrate or protein and, of course, is more fattening.

Fat comes mainly from meats and dairy products but can also be found in high quantities in some baked goods, salad dressings, chips, fries, and candy bars. In countries where individuals eat more fruits, vegetables, chicken, and fish—for example, in Greece, Italy, France, Spain, some Caribbean Islands, and many parts of South America and Asia—obesity is relatively rare but is increasing. Some of the oldest individuals in the world live in Greece and Japan. It also is interesting that in laboratory experiments when limited amount of food is given to rats, they live about 40% longer than when they are allowed to eat unlimited quantities of food; furthermore, monkeys also live longer when the amount of food they usually eat is reduced. There is evidence that a low-calorie diet even prolongs the lifespan of old mice by more than 40%. **"Lean and less" is better for humans and animals.** When food is restricted, body temperature and insulin blood levels are lowered and the blood level of a steroid hormone remains steady—these characteristics are found in men who live the longest.

Recent surveys of adults in China reveal that heart disease there is skyrocketing; stroke remains about twice as common as heart attack. About 30% of the Chinese population have hypertension, 33% high cholesterol, 6% diabetes, and another 7% a tendency to develop diabetes. The cause of this unfortunate increase in heart disease apparently is linked to the high prevalence of cigarette smoking, less exercise, and the increasing consumption of animal fats and fast foods, which were unavailable until recently (it is reported that one American fast-food chain now has 430 restaurants in China). These trends in disease and unhealthy lifestyles are spreading to many developing countries.

Some individuals who are compulsive eaters apparently derive gratification in eating excessively. Eating offers a comfort zone that relieves tension and anxiety. Many of these individuals may have emotional problems that are temporarily alleviated by excess food consumption. In these persons, the compulsive desire to eat may be viewed as somewhat similar to the chronic alcoholic or the smoker who becomes addicted to nicotine in cigarettes. Weight continues to increase, and some become morbidly obese, meaning that they have gained as much or more than twice their normal healthy weight. Obesity of this magnitude is a deadly condition that often results in the individual being immobilized and bedridden because of the extreme effort and difficulty in walking or even changing positions. Very few hospitals have large enough wheelchairs, hospital beds, stretchers, operating tables, gowns, blood pressure cuffs, weighing scales, or MRI and CAT machines to accommodate these markedly obese individuals. Furthermore, excess fat frequently prevents MRI or CAT scan images from being clear enough to see any injured areas or other abnormalities; excess breast fat may also interfere with accurate interpretation of mammograms. Even the average door width is often too narrow for the morbidly obese to pass through. These limitations and immobility add further to the frustration, humiliation, depression, and misery of these unfortunate individuals. Most individuals with morbid obesity develop hypertension, diabetes, and elevated harmful fats in their blood, and they die at a relatively young age from heart or kidney disease or stroke. Surgical procedures, which limit the amount of food absorbed from the intestinal tract, may be needed to help lose weight and for survival of some morbidly obese individuals. It is estimated that more than 100,000 morbidly obese Americans underwent these surgical procedures in 2004—about four times as many as in 1998.

Combating obesity in these individuals is extremely difficult. Special clinics exist to provide dietary treatment and emotional support to groups of these patients, which seems more effective than working with individual patients. Drugs that reduce the desire to eat or decrease the amount of fat absorbed from the intestine may be tried but usually are not very helpful and may cause undesirable side effects. Such drugs should be used only under the direction of a physician and should be used in conjunction with a healthy diet and regular exercise. **Dietary supplements and products containing ephedra (ma huang), or ephedrine, or phenylpropanolamine for weight loss should never be used because they can stimulate the nervous system and cause a marked increase in blood pressure and heart rate and may occasionally cause a heart attack, stroke, and death.** Initially, the American Medical Association and the American Heart Association urged that all ephedra supplements be banned; it was then banned by the National Football League, and its use by athletes in college competition and in the Olympics was prohibited. Unfortunately, professional baseball, basketball, and hockey teams did not make every effort to prevent the serious health consequences of this very dangerous drug. However, in December 2003, the Food and Drug Administration (FDA) announced that the sale of supplements containing ephedra would become unlawful.

Ephedra probably played a role in the death of 23-year-old Baltimore Orioles pitcher, Steve Bechler, who collapsed during a workout and died the next day. 100 deaths have been reported in persons taking ephedra, and numerous episodes of brain damage (strokes), seizures, heat stroke, heart attack, and mental changes (psychosis) have been reported.

Other supplements are available that are supposed to increase metabolism and burn fat. An article in *The New York Times* in March 2003 recounted the frightening experience of Jennifer Rosenthal, a 28-year-old California mother. She was not overweight but "just wanted to stay in shape." A friend recommended that she take capsules (containing usnic acid) that were supposed to increase metabolism and burn off fat. In early October she started taking half the maximum dose of the capsules; about a month later, she was in a coma, on a respirator, and her skin was a dusky yellow. Fortunately, a liver from a cadaver became available and was transplanted to replace her own severely damaged liver, which had shrunk to about one third of its normal size. Without this transplant she would have died in a few days. Currently, she is taking many medications, some of which are essential to prevent rejection of the transplanted liver. She will have to continue some medications for the rest of her life, and she must limit many of her activities forever.

It is extremely important to appreciate that some dietary supplements (products of herbs and plants) may be very harmful or fatal. Unfortunately, these substances are not regulated and are easily obtainable in food stores and over the Internet. You should never use a supplement if its safety and effectiveness are unknown. It is always wise to ask a physician when considering the use of a supplement.

Former U.S. Surgeon General David Satcher stated, "Being overweight or obese may soon cause as much preventable disease and death as tobacco," and Dr. Mark Jacobsen of the American Academy of Pediatrics has suggested that the cost of obesity-related diseases may outstrip the healthcare costs of cigarette smoking. American physicians, although rarely obese themselves, are aware of the dangerous consequences of obesity, and they should strive to educate their patients about its seriousness. More attention should be paid to educating physicians, medical students, and other healthcare providers regarding the importance of proper nutrition, exercise, and weight control for their patients. Furthermore, the government and local communities can be helpful in raising the level of awareness of the serious health risks of obesity. Educating the public about the seriousness of obesity and related diseases that can be prevented, or at least controlled, is essential and may save many lives. It is very difficult or impossible to get individuals to lose weight if they are not motivated to do so. However, parental involvement may be especially helpful in influencing some obese children and teenagers to eat healthy food and to exercise adequately. High-fat and high-sugar foods—cookies, candy, potato or corn chips, doughnuts, bakery products, crackers, sodas, and ice cream—should not be readily available. Even low-fat foods usually have a significant amount of calories. A parent's example and effort to help a child cope with any problem can sometimes be the key to success.

Americans spend $30 billion each year trying to become and remain slim through various diets and exercise programs. Unfortunately, of those individuals who lose weight, 95% regain the pounds they lost! This does not mean than one should not attempt to lose weight. **Fortunately, modest weight loss of even 10 pounds or 10% of body weight may lower blood pressure, blood sugar, and cholesterol. The efforts of teachers, parents, and the community should focus on *prevention* of obesity by introducing healthy lifestyles to preschool children and those in kindergarten, first and second grade and then reinforcing, expanding, and promoting healthy lifestyle in all grades through high school.**

The Best Eating Plan

- Maintain a weight near the standard acceptable range (Table 1) to prevent becoming overweight or underweight.
- Include foods (particularly lots of fruits and vegetables—fresh, frozen, canned, or dried) that are high in potassium (which tends to lower blood pressure and prevent strokes), other minerals, and fiber.
- Limit the percentage of daily calories from dietary fat to 30% or less and especially decrease saturated fat to 10% or less.
- Include low-fat or nonfat dairy foods—major sources of calcium and protein.
- Limit the amount of meat and poultry to no more than two 3-ounce servings daily. Eating a variety of fish as a major source of protein is recommended; however, fish that may contain mercury (particularly fatty fish, e.g., swordfish, shark, king mackerel, tilefish, and albacore tuna) should be limited to no more that once weekly and should be avoided by pregnant women or women of childbearing age. Although shellfish, such as shrimp and lobster, have a moderate amount of cholesterol, they have very little fat and are low in calories; they may be eaten occasionally if they are not prepared or soaked with butter. Avoid fried fish and poultry, especially batter dipped or breaded.
- Limit sugar and "junk" foods (sodas, chips, candy bars, etc.) that are high in calories and low in nutritional value.
- Help lower elevated blood pressure by limiting total salt intake to no more than 6 grams (about 1 teaspoonful) daily (equivalent to 2,400 milligrams of sodium). The 1 teaspoon would include salt in processed food and salt used in cooking and at the table.
- Limit alcohol consumption to no more than 2 drinks of wine, beer, or spirits per day for men (1 drink per day for women).
- Help lower the amounts of "bad" (LDL) cholesterol and triglyceride (fat) in the blood, if they are elevated, by decreasing the amount of dietary fat to 30% and saturated fat to 10% or less of total calories and by decreasing cholesterol consumption.
- Eat foods high in fiber, such as whole-grain cereals and breads,

fruits, vegetables, and legumes (beans and lentils). Fiber is a complex carbohydrate and provides no calories because it is not digested by the body. Fiber appears to play a beneficial role in reducing the risk of heart disease, diabetes, and colon and breast cancer. It is recommended that adults try to eat about 25 to 30 grams daily; children should aim for 5 grams plus their age in grams. Fruits and vegetables and their skins (if edible) are a particularly abundant and healthy source of fiber.

- Help lower elevated blood sugar by limiting carbohydrates, especially sweets and sugar.

Carbohydrates provide the major energy source for the body, and they consist of two types: complex (starch) and simple (sugar). The body converts these to glucose, which provides energy. Glucose is especially important for brain function. Complex carbohydrates are abundant in breads, pastas, rice, potatoes, and vegetables, whereas sweet-tasting foods usually contain simple carbohydrate, that is, sugar found in candy, cookies, ice cream, sodas, fruits, and dairy products.

The consumption of adequate dietary calcium (up to 1,500 milligrams daily for adults, but the requirement depends on age and gender) and adequate vitamin D (usually about 400 IU daily; some vitamin D is produced in the skin by exposure to sunlight, but older persons and those not exposed to sunlight may require 800 IU) helps your body absorb calcium. A blood test can determine whether you have adequate vitamin D in your body. Both calcium and vitamin D are important in preventing and treating osteoporosis. Some fruit juice, milk, and foods are fortified with calcium and vitamin D; however, supplemental calcium and vitamin D may be needed. Additional calcium and vitamin D should not be consumed by those who have had calcium stones in their urinary tract.

Adequate vitamins and minerals are essential for health. Although the body cannot make vitamins (A, C, D, E, K, B_6, B_{12}, thiamin,

The Best Eating Plan

riboflavin, niacin, folic acid, biotin, and pantothenic acid) or minerals (sodium, potassium, calcium, magnesium, manganese, copper, iodine, fluoride, iron, phosphorus, selenium, molybdenum, and zinc), severe deficiencies of these substances are uncommon in the United States if people are in good health and are eating a balanced diet with a variety of nutritious foods. However, many adults, particularly older persons who are chronically ill and those who do not eat a balanced diet, may have a mild deficiency of some vitamins, especially vitamins D and B_{12}. It is estimated that 40% of the U.S. population does not consume adequate folic acid. It is recommended that women of childbearing age consume 400 micrograms of folic acid daily (which is contained in most multivitamin pills), since this can markedly decrease development of a certain type of nerve defect in their babies. Folic acid can also be beneficial by reducing homocysteine in the blood, since homocysteine may contribute to hardening of the arteries. Therefore, it seems reasonable to take a one-a-day vitamin to avoid a vitamin deficiency. Megadoses of vitamins should be avoided because some of them can cause serious side effects. There is no convincing evidence that large doses of vitamin C can prevent infections, cancer, or any other disease. High doses of vitamin C may sometimes cause kidney stones. A high intake of vitamin A has been associated with an increased risk of hip fracture in postmenopausal women and with fetal abnormalities during early pregnancy. Very high doses of vitamin A and beta carotene may increase the occurrence of lung cancer (particularly in smokers and workers exposed to asbestos) and may also increase death from heart and blood vessel damage.

Individuals on crash or fad diets and strict vegetarians can develop vitamin and mineral deficiencies, which require adding appropriate amounts of the deficient vitamins and/or minerals. Crash or fad diets should not be used to lose weight because they can be hazardous to your health. Increased consumption of some minerals can be dangerous and should never be taken without the recommendation of a physician.

Finally, it is important for menstruating women to consume adequate dietary iron to avoid the possibility of an iron-deficiency anemia. Pregnant women should follow the diet prescribed by their healthcare provider. Breastfeeding appears to have a protective effect against the development of obesity in the offspring. Also, mothers who breastfeed may return to prepregnancy weight more quickly than those who bottlefeed their babies.

It is especially important to read food labels and become aware of foods that have a high concentration of total fat, saturated fat, cholesterol, sugar, and sodium so that you can limit them.

Elevated bad cholesterol (LDL) levels and probably elevated triglyceride (another fat) levels in the blood increase the risk of heart attacks, strokes, and hardening of the arteries. In the presence of hypertension, the risk of these complications is significantly greater, which makes it even more important to reduce the level of these bad fats in addition to normalizing blood pressure.

In addition to reducing the fat in your diet to lower bad cholesterol and triglyceride

- Limit refined sugar in the diet to help reduce elevated triglyceride.
- Reduce excess weight to a healthy range (see Table 1).
- Take cholesterol- and lipid (fat)-lowering drugs if your physician indicates.

Be aware of foods that contain cholesterol and harmful fats, particularly saturated fats and trans-fats. However, be aware that

foods claiming to be low fat may be high in calories and undesirable for those trying to lose weight.

Harmful Cholesterol (LDL)

These are found in foods of animal origin. Foods high in cholesterol include

- Meats
- Organ meats
- Egg yolks
- Shellfish
- Dairy products and products made with whole milk (butter, ice cream, whipping cream, heavy cream, half-and-half, cheese, yogurt)

Low-fat or fat-free dairy products have less cholesterol.

Because your body makes adequate cholesterol, you should limit consumption to less than 300 milligrams a day. Cholesterol does not provide calories, but increased amounts of cholesterol and LDL can damage and clog arteries.

Saturated Fats

These raise the bad cholesterol (LDL) and increase the risk of heart attack and stroke. They include

- Animal fats such as lard and full-fat dairy products
- Chocolate, cocoa (cocoa powder is acceptable)
- Coconut and palm oil (often used in baked products)
- Some vegetable shortening

Trans-Fats (Trans-Fatty Acids)

Trans-fats are also saturated fats artificially prepared by adding hydrogen to vegetable oils to solidify the oil and increase its shelf life (very little trans-fats occur naturally). They are even more unhealthy and harmful than naturally occurring saturated fats, and they increase the risk of heart attack and stroke. They increase bad cholesterol and triglyceride in the blood. They decrease good cholesterol (HDL) in the blood. Trans-fats are often used to make

- French fries
- Chips that are fried
- Tortillas
- Pudding
- Doughnuts
- Crackers
- Multigrain cereal bars
- Cookies and bakery products
- All pie crusts
- Nondairy creamer
- Margarines
- Shortening

The FDA recently announced that food labels will soon include trans-fats. In the mean time, limit saturated fats and foods that are labeled "hydrogenated" or "partially hydrogenated" because the product contains trans-fats. A rough estimate of trans-fats in food can be calculated by subtracting the grams of each fat in the food from the total grams of fat.

Monounsaturated Fats

Whenever possible, replace trans-fats with monounsaturated fats, such as olive, peanut, and canola oil, and avocados. **These are**

extremely healthy fats that tend to lower bad cholesterol (LDL) and do not damage arteries. People in Spain, France, Italy, and Greece who tend to consume fat in the form of olive oil and eat lots of vegetables, fruits, whole grains, and smaller portions of meat and processed foods (known as the "Mediterranean diet") have relatively little heart disease.

Polyunsaturated Fats

These fats include corn, sunflower, safflower, cotton seed, soybean oils, and omega-3 fats (in fish and soy foods), which are also far healthier than saturated fats and may lower bad (LDL) cholesterol. Nevertheless, they can undergo changes in the body that can damage arteries; also, excessive use of any oil can add significant calories and promote weight gain. **If weight loss (when indicated) and diet do not sufficiently lower the bad cholesterol (LDL) and triglyceride, then medication may be necessary.**

Limiting the percentage of protein in your diet is not recommended for weight reduction. A healthy diet should contain 15% to 20% protein. The Atkins diet actually increases protein up to 30% of the diet to replace the marked reduction of carbohydrate; however, a diet that is high in protein can be detrimental to persons with some kidney or liver diseases. Protein is an important source of energy and is essential to build muscles and organs of the body. It is plentiful in many foods, especially meats, poultry, fish, shell fish, nuts, dairy foods, eggs, and beans. However, it is best to eat less meat and to trim and remove as much fat from beef, lamb, veal, venison, and pork as possible; skin of poultry should be removed and not eaten because it contains a lot of fat and cholesterol. An egg yolk may contain up to 300 milligrams of cholesterol, that is, the most one should consume daily. Egg whites contain only protein (as do egg beaters) and are very nutritious. Soy foods come in many forms and are a rich source of protein that may lower bad (LDL) cholesterol in the blood.

The Dietary Approaches to Stop Hypertension (DASH) diet (Table 3) has been found to lower blood pressure effectively in hypertensive individuals and to reduce the occurrence of stroke. This diet has also been recommended as an *extremely healthy diet for all Americans*. It has been recommended by the American Heart Association, the National Cancer Institute, the National High Blood Pressure Education Program, the medical profession and registered dietitians. The foods included in the DASH diet are healthy, tasty, and can be easily prepared. The DASH diet is low in fat (about 27% of calories) and has lots of fruits and vegetables (4 to 5 servings of each daily), low-fat or nonfat dairy products, and whole grains, and it effectively lowers bad cholesterol. Nuts, seeds, and legumes (peas, beans, and lentils) provide healthy protein, allowing smaller amounts of meat, fish, and poultry. Health and nutrition experts agree that the DASH diet is the healthiest diet ever recommended!

In one study, after 8 weeks on the DASH diet, the systolic and diastolic pressures in hypertensive individuals decreased by 11.4 and 5.5 mm Hg, respectively. Even persons with high normal blood pressures experienced a decrease of about 3.5 mm Hg in their diastolic pressure. On the other hand, researchers did not observe any change in blood pressure of individuals on the typical American diet, which contains approximately 37% of calories in the form of fat and is low in fruits and vegetables. **The decrease in blood pressure found with the DASH diet occurred without any other lifestyle changes, which indicates the value of decreasing fat and increasing consumption of fruits and vegetables. A second study showed that by further decreasing dietary salt, the blood pressure was lowered even more.**

Experimental and clinical studies indicate that increased consumption of potassium is helpful in gradually reducing blood pressure and preventing stroke. Because of increased emphasis on fruits, vegetables, and nuts, seeds, and legumes (e.g., peas, beans,

The Best Eating Plan

43

Table 3   The DASH Diet (Based on about 2,000 Calories Per Day)

Food Group	Daily Servings	Serving Sizes	Examples	Significance to the DASH Diet
Grains and grain products	7–8	1 slice bread ½ cup dry cereal ½ cup cooked rice, pasta, or cereal	Whole-wheat bread, (1/2) English muffin, (small) pita bread, bagel, cereals, grits, oatmeal (typical bagel = 4 servings of grains)	Major sources of energy and fiber
Vegetables	4–5	1 cup raw leafy vegetable ½ cup cooked vegetable 6 oz vegetable juice	Tomatoes, potatoes, carrots, peas, squash, broccoli, turnip greens, collards, kale, spinach, artichokes, beans, sweet potatoes	Rich sources of potassium, magnesium, and fiber
Fruits	4–5	6 oz fruit juice 1 medium fruit ¼ cup dried fruit ½ cup fresh, frozen, or canned fruit	Apricots, bananas, dates, oranges, grapefruit, mangoes, melons, peaches, pineapples, prunes, raisins, strawberries, tangerines	Important sources of potassium, magnesium, and fiber
Low-fat or nonfat dairy foods	2–3	8 oz milk 1 cup yogurt 1½ oz cheese	Skim or 1% milk, skim or low-fat buttermilk, nonfat or low-fat yogurt, part-skim mozzarella cheese, nonfat cheese	Major sources of calcium and protein
Meats, poultry, fish	2 or less	3 oz cooked meats, poultry, or fish	Select only lean meat; trim away visible fats; broil, roast, or boil instead of frying; remove skin from poultry (can also grill)	Rich sources of protein and magnesium
*Eggs	No more than 3 per week	One egg or two egg whites		

Nuts, seeds, legumes	4–5 per week	1½ oz or ⅓ cup nuts, ½ oz or 2 tablespoons seeds, ½ cup cooked legumes	(Unsalted) almonds, filberts, mixed nuts, peanuts, walnuts, sunflower seeds, kidney beans, lentils	Rich sources of energy, magnesium, potassium, protein, and fiber
Fats and oils	2–3	1 tsp soft margarine, 1 Tbsp low-fat mayonnaise, 2 Tbsp light salad dressing, 1 tsp vegetable oil	Soft margarine, low-fat mayonnaise, light salad dressing, vegetable oil, (such as olive, corn, canola, or safflower)	DASH has 27% of calories as fat, including that in or added to foods
Sweets	5 per week	1 Tbsp sugar, 1 Tbsp jelly or jam, ½ oz jelly beans, 8 oz lemonade	Maple syrup, sugar, jelly, jam, fruit-flavored gelatin, jelly beans, hard candy, fruit punch, sorbet, ices	Sweets should be low in fat

Source: "Dietary Approaches to Stop Hypertension" (DASH). The Sixth Report of the Joint National Committee (November 1997). The diet is rich in fruits, vegetables, and low-fat dairy foods and low in cholesterol, total, and saturated fat. It is high in fiber, potassium, calcium, and magnesium and moderately high in protein. (The DASH Diet—NIH publication 01-4082. Revised May 2001.) Slight modifications in parentheses for clarity.

*Added to DASH diet. Note: count eggs in recipes; egg whites do not have to be limited.

lentils, soy beans), the potassium content of the DASH diet is roughly 2.5 times that consumed in an ordinary diet in the United States. The roles played by other minerals in fruits and vegetables (such as calcium and magnesium) and by fat reduction in decreasing blood pressure are less clear. It appears that some salt-sensitive hypertensives who are calcium-deficient may lower their blood pressure by consuming foods high in calcium, which may increase salt and water excretion. The DASH diet may actually prevent hypertension in some individuals, and it is an extremely healthy diet that all Americans should follow. For individuals with high blood pressure, however, salt should be limited to 6 grams (1 teaspoonful) daily instead of the 7.5 grams used in the DASH diet. For those who are lactose intolerant and for those who have trouble digesting dairy products and milk, lactose-free milk or milk pretreated with lactase enzyme can be used. Also, lactase drops (available at grocery or drug stores) can be added to dairy products, or lactase pills can be taken to prevent indigestion so that these high-calcium foods can still be enjoyed. Calcium-fortified orange and other juices, soy or rice milk, are other alternative sources of calcium.

The benefits of the foods recommended in the DASH diet are particularly compelling arguments for adhering to this diet whether your weight is in a healthy range or above it. For example, increasing consumption of fruits and vegetables, which contain beneficial chemicals called antioxidants, may protect you from various cancers, heart disease, hypertension, and stroke. Whole-grain foods may also protect from cancer, heart disease, stroke, and diabetes. Calcium-rich foods can protect from osteoporosis and possibly colon cancer. Frequently eating fish may decrease the chance of heart attack and lower blood pressure. Nuts are a healthy type of fat and protein, but they are high in calories and should only be eaten in recommended amounts. **The DASH diet is an excellent diet for individuals with type 2 diabetes, but foods that are high in sugar or refined carbohydrate, fruits, and grains**

should be limited. However, if you are a diabetic, it is best to consult a physician or registered dietitian about the exact composition of your diet.

Lean meat and poultry in no more than two servings a day of 3 ounces (about the size of a deck of cards) per serving will lower the fat and calories you consume. Including fish in your diet (especially fish with omega-3 fats such as salmon, halibut, tuna, mackerel, and herring at least 2 times per week) is heart healthy. **Sugar and foods high in sugar can be eaten occasionally, and whole grains should take the place of foods made with refined (white) flour (such as bread, bagels, crackers, and rolls).** Avoiding foods high in saturated fats is most important. Butter or margarine with trans-fats should be avoided or replaced with Benecol (a butter-like substance that can lower cholesterol), soft or whipped (tub-variety) margarine, or Smart Balance, which has no trans-fats. **However, these high-caloric butter substitutes should be used sparingly if you are trying to lose weight.** Likewise, monounsaturated fats (e.g., olive or canola oil or omega 3-fats in fish) are particularly healthful but are high in calories just as other fats are; thus, stick with the recommended amounts. Another alternative is to choose "fruit butters" such as apple butter, which does not actually contain fat but is a fruit spread. Choose fruit butters that do not have added sugar.

Good strategies to help you eat healthy include the following:

- Use a smaller plate when eating so that you put less food on your plate.
- Avoid second helpings.
- Bake, broil, steam, grill, boil, sauté (in broth, olive oil, or non-stick spray), poach, or roast. **Avoid frying**.
- Drink a glass of water before eating a meal so that you feel full. Low-calorie soups with meals will also help make you feel full;

however, most soups contain lots of salt, and individuals trying to reduce consumption of sodium may have to limit soups in their diet. Reduced sodium soups are now available.

- Divide your plate into three sections for (1) starch (grains); (2) fish, poultry, or meat; and (3) vegetables and/or fruits. By doing this, you can control portion sizes and avoid overeating (see **Figure 6**).
- If you snack between meals, choose healthy snacks, such as one fresh fruit, one-half cup cut vegetables with salsa, 3-cups unsalted popcorn (air popped with no fat added or low-fat microwave popcorn), two rice cakes, four slices melba toast, three graham crackers, 1 cup of low-fat yogurt, and diet gelatin.
- Increase consumption of fruits at breakfast and in place of high-caloric desserts.
- Learn which foods to choose and limit (see **Table 4**).

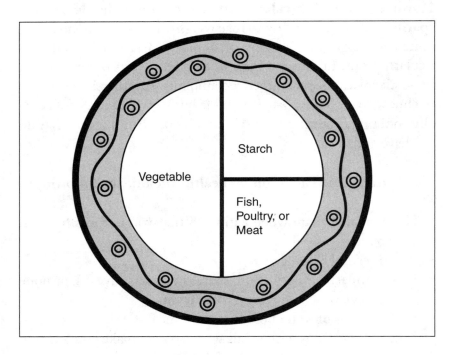

Figure 6 Your dinner plate (10.5-inch diameter).

Table 4 Some Foods to Choose or Limit

Food Groups	Foods to Choose	Foods to Limit
Grains, Starches	Whole-grain breads and cereals, rice cakes, whole-grain crackers, pasta, brown rice, hot and cold cereals (with no added sugar), corn, sweet and white potatoes	Doughnuts, Danish, croissants, biscuits, refined muffins, sugary cereals, French toast, crackers made with fat, granola-type cereals, butter or cheese sauce, stuffing, fried potatoes, fried rice, French fries
Fruits and Vegetables	Fresh, frozen or canned fruits (in water not syrup), fresh or frozen vegetables, dried fruits, fruit and vegetable juices (without added sugar and low in sodium)	Coconut, fried vegetables, prepared or packaged foods in cream, butter, oil or cheese sauce
Dairy Products	Skim milk, 1% or fat-free milk, skim buttermilk, nonfat and low-fat yogurt and cottage cheese, low-fat cheeses (containing no more than 3 grams of fat per serving)	2% and whole milk, buttermilk, cream, half-and-half, cheeses made from whole milk and cream, whole milk cottage cheese, whole milk ricotta, mozzarella or imitation hard cheeses, sour cream, heavy and whipping cream, regular yogurt
Fish, Poultry, Meat, Eggs	Fish, shellfish, tuna packed in water, chicken and turkey without skin, lean cuts of beef, lamb, veal or pork, venison, egg yolks (limit to 3 or less a week), egg substitute, egg whites	Prime-grade fatty cuts of beef, fast-food hamburgers, lamb or pork, ribs, bacon, sausage, duck, goose, regular cold cuts, hot dogs, tuna packed in oil, organ meats, ham hocks, fast-food chicken nuggets
Nuts, Seeds, Legumes	Unsalted nuts and seeds, dry or canned (low sodium) lentils, beans, black beans, and peas, soy beans, peanut butter	Prepared canned beans and lentils; salted nuts and seeds
Fats and Oils	Vegetable oils (1 tsp), margarine (1 tsp), diet margarine (1 tbsp); mayonnaise: regular (1 tsp), reduced-fat (1 tbsp); salad dressing: regular (1 tbsp), low-fat (2 tbsp)	Coconut or palm oil (mostly found in baked goods), butter, whipped butter, cream cheese, heavy cream, bacon, sour cream, shortening or lard, high-calorie salad dressings (e.g., containing cheese)

Table 4 (continued)		
Food Groups	Foods to Choose	Foods to Limit
Seasonings, Sweets, and Miscellaneous	All herbs and spices (without salt), pepper, mustard, low-sodium ketchup, vinegar, hot sauce, salsa, lemon or lime juice, low-sodium soy sauce, chili sauce, sorbet, nonfat ice cream and frozen yogurt, flavored ices, angel food cake, fig bars, graham crackers, meringues, pudding made with skim milk, cocoa powder, plain popcorn, low-sodium pretzels, hard candy, jelly beans, maple syrup, jelly, jams, gelatin	Barbecue sauce, cream sauces, cheese sauces, cakes, cookies, pies and pastries, ice cream, chocolate, regular pudding, milkshakes, buttered popcorn, potato chips, pickles, and other fried snacks such as corn chips or tortilla chips

Fruits and vegetables that are deeply colored are particularly rich sources of substances (e.g., lycopenes, carotenes, and antioxidants) that may protect against cancer, heart disease, blood clots, cataracts, and macular degeneration (which can cause blindness).

Some Tips on Losing Weight

1. Losing excess weight requires, above all, determination and persistence. Some may find it especially helpful to lose weight with a friend or a group of individuals who are also trying to lose weight. "Weight Watchers" encourages groups of overweight individuals to work together to lose weight mainly by reducing the amount of calories they eat, rather than by following a particular diet. Increased physical activity is also emphasized. Some find this approach very helpful; however, many do not adhere to this program, and most regain any weight they lose. There are no magic diets or pills. There are all sorts of special diets that often make fraudulent and unscientific claims of how these diets can dramatically reduce weight. **However, the fact that 95% of persons who lose weight then regain it indicates that special diets are not the answer. So-called crash or fad diets that produce very rapid**

weight loss by severe caloric restriction can be dangerous for some. High-fat diets may be harmful to patients with high blood cholesterol levels, atherosclerosis (hardening of the arteries), diabetes, or poor kidney or liver function.

It is beyond the scope of this book to discuss the many weight-loss diets that are aggressively marketed throughout the United States. However, popular weight-loss diets, proposed by the late Dr. Robert Atkins, Dr. Dean Ornish, Mr. Robert Pritikin, Dr. Arthur Agatston, Dr. Barry Sears, and Mr. Leighton Steward, should be mentioned. These diets differ remarkably in their composition, and controversy continues regarding which is preferable and whether any of these diets should be recommended for weight reduction. All of these weight-loss programs recommend moderate exercise in addition to the various diets.

The Atkins diet consists of a high-protein, high-fat, and low-carbohydrate diet (60% fat, about 10% carbohydrate, and 25% to 30% protein). Metabolizing or burning up body fat on this low-carbohydrate diet produces chemicals called ketones, which suppress appetite and sometimes cause nausea, fatigue, and a sweet breath odor. Dr. Atkins believed firmly that foods that markedly elevate blood sugar (these are called high glycemic foods) and thereby stimulate insulin release from the pancreas play the major role in weight gain. These foods were said to increase hunger and not suppress the desire to eat. Reports indicate that 50 million Americans have tried a low-carbohydrate diet, such as the Atkins diet. Furthermore, a number of Atkins grocery items are being sold in a variety of food outlets, and Friday's chain restaurants are working with the Atkins organization to produce low-carbohydrate foods for their members. The currently popular high-fat/low-carbohydrate Atkins diet apparently causes a greater weight loss for 6 months than a low-fat/high-carbohydrate diet; however, after 1 year, weight loss was not significantly different from a calorie-controlled low-fat diet. In one study, about 40% did not stay on the Atkins diet.

The Best Eating Plan

The Atkins diet should not be used by those with impaired kidney or liver function because it may aggravate kidney failure or liver disease. Furthermore, as Atkins indicates, the diet should not be used during pregnancy or when mothers are nursing. Although in the short-run this diet may decrease blood cholesterol levels in some, cholesterol levels may become significantly elevated; its effects on heart health, cancer, and diabetes are unclear. This diet limits consumption of fruits and vegetables, a rich source of antioxidants, which are important in preventing and combating a variety of diseases. The original Atkins diet did not make a distinction between "good" and "bad" fat, and the diet permitted consumption of both. However, more recently, because of years of scientific criticism, representatives of Atkins have altered the original Atkins diet program that permitted consumption of unlimited fat and red meat. They now recommend smaller portions of meat and limiting saturated fat, which mainly is present in meat, cheese, butter, and shortening, to 20%; the remaining fat should be mainly from vegetable oil and fish. Although this revision is healthier than the original Atkins diet, it is still considerably higher in fat than most of the medical profession and nutritionists recommend. The link between a high-fat diet and hardening of the arteries and colon cancer is compelling, and there is recent evidence that excess cholesterol in the diet may increase the risk of Alzheimer's disease. Prolonged consumption of high-fat foods can damage arteries in the heart and brain and cause heart disease and stroke. Furthermore, prolonged consumption of a high-protein diet may increase loss of calcium from bone, which is undesirable, especially in those with decreased bone calcium or osteoporosis.

The recent emphasis on the importance of eating low-carbohydrate diets is unfortunate and misleading; it is not the answer to losing weight. Recent scientific studies have shown that you can lose weight on a high-carbohydrate diet, as long as you consume complex carbohydrates (e.g., whole-grain foods, fruits, vegetables, legumes, breads, cereals, brown rice, and whole-wheat pastas). Complex carbohydrates are highly nutritious and have a relatively low-glycemic index (i.e., they do not increase blood sugar very much); they can be consumed in large amounts without causing weight gain. On the other hand, simple carbohydrates (e.g., sugar, sweets, white bread, white rice, and potatoes) are low in nutrients and have a high-glycemic index, and their consumption should be limited.

The term *net carb* has been used by some to indicate the amount of a carbohydrate that is absorbed from the intestine and may elevate sugar and insulin levels in the blood; however, the amount absorbed from various carbohydrates is not well established, and the term does not help those trying to lose weight. The FDA and nutritionists do not recognize net carbohydrate figures.

Ornish prescribes a very low-fat, high-carbohydrate diet (10% to 15% fat, greater than 65% carbohydrate, and 10% to 20% protein). The Ornish diet avoids simple and refined carbohydrates (e.g., sugar, white flour, and white bread) but advocates carbohydrates in their whole or complex forms (e.g., beans, brown rice, whole grains, fruits, vegetables, nuts, and unrefined whole-wheat bread), which also are rich in antioxidants and fiber. Fiber slows absorption in the intestine of these complex carbohydrates and also may decrease the chances of developing colon cancer. Some individuals may find it difficult to adhere to a diet so low in fat for an extended period of time. A low-fat diet is not recommended for children under 2 years of age because at a young age the nervous system requires adequate fat for normal development. There are no long-term concerns with a very low-fat diet; however, a very high-carbohydrate diet should be avoided in individuals with adult-onset diabetes.

The Pritikin weight-loss program, developed by Robert Pritikin and his father, Nathan, is in many ways similar to the Ornish diet program. It emphasizes limiting fat, choosing the right carbohydrate-

The Best Eating Plan

rich foods that have high fiber (e.g., vegetables, fruits, and un-processed grains), and low-fat dairy products, and also eating fre-quently (to avoid hunger).

Dr. Arthur Agatston's recently publicized "South Beach Diet" is neither a low-fat nor low-carbohydrate diet. He correctly empha-sizes eating balanced meals that contain good fats (monounsatu-rated and polyunsaturated fats such as olive, canola, and peanut oil, low-fat dairy products, and nuts) and good carbohydrates (such as whole-wheat bread, whole-wheat pasta, and most cere-als). He urges avoiding sugar and avoiding or limiting products that are made with white flour (such as white bread and pasta), po-tatoes, and white rice. Usual amounts of lean beef, pork, veal, lamb, chicken, turkey, fish, shellfish, vegetables, and fruits are permitted. Snacks between meals and desserts are also recommended.

The "South Beach Diet" seems reasonably balanced and more palatable than the Atkins or Ornish diets. Dr. Agatston (in agree-ment with Dr. Atkins) emphasizes the importance of limiting foods, especially carbohydrates, that have a high glycemic index, which means that they particularly increase the sugar and insulin levels in the blood. Insulin causes some of the sugar to be stored in muscle and liver and some to be changed into fat. The fact that some foods (especially sugar, white bread, and other products made with white flower, white rice, and potatoes) have a higher glycemic index than others has been known for many years. It makes good sense to avoid or limit foods with a very high glycemic index when trying to lose weight. However, the American Dia-betes Association states that there is not sufficient evidence of the benefits of relying on the glycemic index to recommend its use.

Dr. Barry Sears' Zone Diet suggests that maintaining certain ra-tios of carbohydrate to protein and fat and a balance of insulin and certain other hormones is helpful in losing weight. However, there is no evidence that establishes these claims. Those following this diet will lose weight because it is low in calories and emphasizes vegetables and fruits.

Mr. H. Leighton Steward proposes that cutting sugar (The "Sugar Busters" eating plan) is important for losing weight. However, as has been pointed out, lumping "foods such as potatoes, corn, and carrots with refined sugar in cakes, candies, and sodas goes too far." The diet also encourages eating saturated fat and decreasing vegetable consumption, which will not help one to lose weight.

Furthermore, none of these diets, except the Pritikin diet, mentions the importance of limiting the use of dietary salt, which, as previously discussed, is very important in the prevention and treatment of hypertension. Salt limitation should be recommended in almost every diet. As mentioned previously, in addition to its dietary recommendations, the DASH diet emphasizes the importance of limiting salt consumption. More recently, the principles of the DASH diet have been incorporated into the Mayo Clinic Healthy Weight Pyramid. **The Federal Government, the National Academy of Sciences, and the Center for Science in the Public Interest are also recommending that Americans reduce their salt consumption.**

There are no very long-term studies on the benefits or the effectiveness of any of the popular weight-loss diets. With any special diet, particularly when the goal is weight reduction, it is important to make certain that the diet is nutritionally adequate and that vitamin and mineral deficiencies are avoided. These deficiencies are important to recognize and remedy, particularly for those who reduce food consumption to lose weight. With vegetarian diets, which usually are low in fat and very healthy, care must be taken to ensure adequate intake of non-animal calcium and iron-containing foods. Therefore, dietary supplements of vitamins, calcium, and iron may be needed for some vegetarians and for others on a weight-reduction diet, particularly when calories are limited to

1,200 or less daily. The typical American diet contains about 35% fat, 50% carbohydrate, and 15% protein.

2. To lose weight, you must eat fewer calories than what your body needs, and you should burn more calories through physical activity. It is important to stress that weight loss can be easier with proper diet *and* adequate exercise. Exercise also increases lean body mass (muscle tissue). An increase in lean body mass will increase your metabolism, thereby burning more calories. It can be very helpful to keep initially a diary of everything you eat and drink. Such a record will enable you to identify sources of excess calorie consumption. **Reduction of fat, carbohydrate (especially sugar), and portion size is key. Furthermore, it is most helpful to have a weight-loss program that has support services (a registered dietitian and an exercise therapist) and experts to guide and encourage your efforts and to monitor your diet and weight loss.**

Make changes slowly. Also, eat slowly (this will make you feel fuller), and never take second helpings. Eating a large volume of food is encouraged, if it is low in calories, as it will help make you feel full and curb your appetite. A recently proposed "volumetric" diet to lose weight is based on this strategy. Do not skip meals. Skipping meals will not reduce weight, as excess calories are often added to other meals. Furthermore, there is good evidence that skipping breakfast can reduce concentration and performance—especially in schoolwork. A slow, gradual weight loss of 1 to 2 pounds weekly adds up to a significant loss over time. Weigh yourself once a week. Do not be discouraged if you lose more weight in one week and less in another. Permanent weight loss is not a race. Slow and steady wins the game. Many studies show that **rapid weight loss** is typically followed by regaining lost weight.

3. The DASH diet in Table 3 is a balanced and nutritious diet equivalent to 2,000 calories. Highly acclaimed by care

providers, it is the healthiest of all diets. The calories your body burns each day depend on your weight and physical activity. The amount of calories burned also depends on the muscular composition of the body. Individuals with more muscle burn more calories. Using the DASH diet with a reduction in calories and increasing physical activity for a prolonged period are excellent ways to reduce overweight or obesity, lower elevated blood pressure, and decrease harmful blood fats. **Figure 7 displays a proposed pyramid for the DASH diet. This pyramid differs from other well-known pyramids by emphasizing more servings of fruits and vegetables and less consumption of meat, poultry, and fish. However, the recently proposed Mayo Clinic Healthy Weight Pyramid is quite similar and permits consumption of unlimited amounts of healthy fruits and vegetables, as there is only a small amount of calories in large amounts of most of these nutritious foods.** The types of food consumed by individuals of different ethnic, religious, social background, and financial status may vary considerably. However, the number of servings of any food depends on its food group as shown in the DASH pyramid (**Figure 7**).

A balanced diet includes:

- **Moderate food consumption and proper calorie intake for body size and physical activity**
- **An emphasis on plant rather than animal foods**
- **A variety of foods from different food groups to ensure adequate vitamins and minerals. Keeping a record of the food and calories you consume each day can be a very helpful guide**

The DASH diet is extremely healthy for everyone, including those with type 2 diabetes. The main concern with diabetic individuals is almost always the need to reduce excess weight. The DASH diet can effectively reduce hypertension, strokes, overweight, elevated blood fats, and homocysteine (a substance in the blood that may increase hardening of the arteries). This diet also improves the

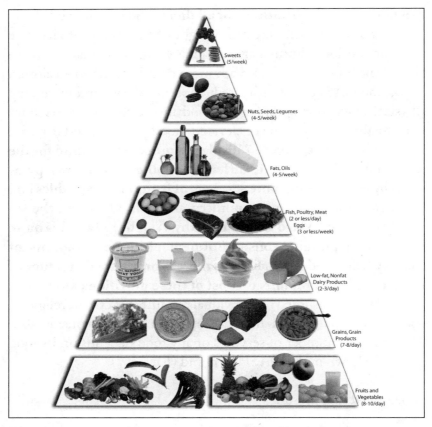

Figure 7 A proposed DASH pyramid. Examples of food groups, serving sizes, and significance to the diet is indicated in Table 3.

action of insulin in diabetics, and if modified to limit sugar and carbohydrate consumption, it can improve diabetes and weight control. It is a uniquely heart-healthy and stroke-preventive diet and, as mentioned previously, *it is highly endorsed by The American Heart Association, The National Cancer Institute, The National High Blood Pressure Program, the medical profession, and registered dietitians.*

4. **To maintain a healthy weight, the daily requirement of most American women and men is about 1,600 and 2,200 calories, respectively.** Of course, individuals who are physically very active will require more calories than those who are inactive and

sedentary (e.g., 2,200 for women and about 2,800 for men). Normally active teenage males may require up to 2,800 calories and when physically very active may require much more. For normally active teenage females, the caloric requirement is about 2,200, but with strenuous activity, they also require more.

A simple rule in estimating the number of daily calories needed to maintain ideal weight is to:

- Multiply the desirable, healthy, **ideal** body weight (IBW) for your height (see **Table 1**) by 13 if you are **sedentary** (performing little if any exercise). For example, a sedentary person with an ideal weight of 150 pounds requires 1,950 calories (i.e., 13 × 150 = 1,950).
- Multiply IBW by 15 if you are **moderately active** (exercising four to five times a week). For example, a moderately active person with an ideal weight of 150 pounds requires 2,250 calories (i.e., 15 × 150 = 2,250).
- Multiply IBW by 17 if you are **very active** (training or exercising 10 or more hours a week). For example, a very active person with an ideal weight of 150 pounds requires 2,550 calories (i.e., 17 × 150 = 2,550).

Reducing food and/or beverage consumption by 500 calories per day usually results in weight loss of about 1 pound per week. This is most easily done by decreasing the size and number of servings (see Tables 5 and 6) and increasing physical activity. However, fat, sugar, sweets, and snacks especially should be reduced.

In general, diets containing 1,000–1,200 calories per day for women and 1,200–1,600 calories per day for men will usually produce a steady and safe rate of weight loss (1–2 pounds per week), especially if combined with exercise. Very low-caloric diets (less than 800 calories per day) are not recommended without physician supervision. Furthermore, megadoses of vitamins can be harmful and are not recommended.

Table 5 Food Groups, Examples, and Calories	

Fruits and Vegetables Group
The following have about 60 calories/serving:

Fruits

Fresh fruit	1 small to medium piece (whole fruit) or ³/₄ to 1 cup of berries
Canned fruit packed in water or fruit juice	¹/₂ cup
Dried fruit	¹/₄ cup

Vegetables

Raw	2 cups
Cooked vegetables or juice	1 cup

Whole-Grains Group
(including cereals, grains, pasta, breads, crackers, and starchy vegetables)
The following have about 80 calories/serving:

Plain cereal, grain (rice), pasta, or starchy vegetable	¹/₂ cup
Bread products (bread, small roll, one-half English muffin, tortilla)	1 piece or 1 ounce (check label for amount)
Crackers, pretzels, etc.	³/₄ to 1 ounce (check label for amount)

Low-Fat, nonfat Dairy Products
The following have about 90 (nonfat) to 120 (low-fat) calories/serving:

Skim, 1% or 2% milk		1 cup
Fat-free, low-fat buttermilk		1 cup
Plain, nonfat, or low-fat yogurt		³/₄ cup
Artificially sweetened, nonfat or low-fat fruit-favored yogurt		1 cup
Cheeses:	1 gram fat or less/ounce	3 ounces
	3 grams fat or less/ounce	2 ounces
Cottage cheese	nonfat or low-fat	³/₄ cup
Cottage cheese	4.5% fat (check label)	¹/₂ cup

Lean Meats, Poultry, Fish
(lean, trimmed of fat before cooking)
The following have about 110 calories/serving:

Meat	Beef, pork, lamb, veal, game		2 ounces
	luncheon meats	3 grams or less of fat/ounce	2 ounces
		Regular	1 ounce
Poultry	White meat, no skin		3 ounces
	dark meat, no skin		2 ounces
Fish	Fresh or frozen, plain		3 ounces
	tuna, water packed shellfish		3 ounces
Egg	Whole, large		1
	Egg whites		2–3
	Egg substitute		¹/₂ cup

Fats, Oils
The following have about 45 calories/serving:

Vegetable oils (olive, corn, safflower, etc.)	1 teaspoon
Margarine (tub, squeeze or stick)	1 teaspoon
Mayonnaise	1 teaspoon
Salad dressing	1 tablespoon

Nuts, Seeds, Legumes
(beans, peas, lentils, soy beans)
The following have about 100 calories/serving:

Beans, peas, lentils (cooked)		1½ cups
Tofu		1 cup
Peanut butter		2 tablespoons
Tahini paste (Sesame seed paste)		4 teaspoons
Nuts:	Almonds	12 nuts
	mixed peanuts	20 nuts
	pecans, walnuts	8 halves
Seeds:	Pumpkin, sunflower	2 tablespoons

Sweets Group
The following have about 100 calories/serving:

Candy bar	approximately one half of a 1.5 ounce bar
M&Ms	approximately one half of a 1.7 ounce package (about 35 plain M&Ms, 12 peanut M&Ms)
Jelly beans or Lifesavers	10 each
Others (check labels closely)	

Table 4 shows the food groups with examples of various foods to choose and foods to limit. **Table 5** indicates the calories in one serving of food in various food groups. **Table 6** indicates the approximate caloric requirement and servings of each food group for children, teenagers, and adults recommended by the U.S. Department of Agriculture (the number of servings depends on age). However, the **DASH diet emphasizes daily consumption of four to five servings of both fruits and vegetables for adults.**

5. Those who wish to lose weight must recognize the dangers of snacking. A significant problem for individuals who gain weight or become obese is partly due to selecting high-caloric, nonnutritious foods and snacks and poor portion control ("supersizing").

Table 6 How Many Servings Do You Need Each Day?			
(Recommended by the U.S. Department of Agriculture)			
	Children ages 2 to 6 years, women, some older adults (about 1,600 calories)	Older children, teen girls, active women, most men (about 2,200 calories)	Teen boys, active men (about 2,800 calories)
Food Group	Servings	Servings	Servings
Grains Group Bread, cereal, rice, and pasta, especially whole grain	6	9	11
Vegetable Group	3	4	5
Fruit Group	2	3	4
Milk Group Milk, yogurt, and cheese— preferably fat free or low fat	2 or 3*	2 or 3*	2 or 3*
Meat and Beans Group Meat, poultry, fish, dry beans, eggs, and nuts— preferably lean or low fat	2, for a total of 5 ounces	2, for a total of 6 ounces	3, for a total of 7 ounces

Adapted from U.S. Department of Agriculture, Center for Nutrition Policy and Promotion with modifications.

*The number of servings depends on your age. Older children and teenagers (ages 9 to 18 years) and adults over the age of 50 need three servings daily. Others need two servings daily. During pregnancy and lactation, the recommended number of milk group servings is the same as that of nonpregnant women.

Keep portions small. **Doughnuts, Danish pastries, most muffins, cakes, crackers, cookies, chips, and all sorts of candies and sweets are high in fats and/or sugar and calories. These snacks do not have to be totally eliminated, but they can be replaced with fruit and vegetables.** Raw fruit, celery and carrot sticks, broccoli, cauliflower, whole-grain bread, bread sticks, unbuttered and unsalted popcorn, unsalted whole-wheat pretzels, graham crackers, low-fat or fat-free yogurt, and snack crackers (e.g., Finn Crisps and matzoh) contain little or no fat and relatively few calories and may effectively relieve hunger. There is convincing evidence that consumption of dietary fiber, which is especially abundant in vegetables, fruits, whole-grain foods, (e.g., whole-grain breads and cereals, whole-wheat pasta, brown rice, barley, legumes, nuts, and whole-wheat low-fat snack crackers), decreases carbohydrate and fat absorption from the intestine and the risk of weight gain and obesity. The healthiest snacks are fresh fruits and vegetables because they are low in calories and high in nutrition; they have lots of vitamins, minerals, antioxidants (protective chemicals), and fiber.

Whole-grain foods are better than processed grains (e.g., white bread and white rice) because they supply more nutrients and fiber. Fiber is filling and also promotes regular bowel function. Fruit and vegetable juice are very nutritious; however, they do not provide nearly the amount of fiber present in fresh fruit. Vegetable juice also usually contains a very high content of sodium, which is undesirable, whereas fruit juice contains lots of potassium which is beneficial because, as indicated previously, it can lower elevated blood pressure and reduce the risk of a stroke.

6. **Drinking a lot of fluid (eight glasses daily of water or any low-caloric drink) can help curb the urge to snack.** Although milk and fruit juice are healthful, they do contribute easy-to-consume calories. **Whole milk should be replaced with skim or low-fat milk. Fruit juice should be 100% unsweetened and limited to 8 ounces per day, and soda and drinks containing sugar should be avoided and replaced with sugarless diet drinks or noncaloric flavored seltzers.** Use noncaloric sweeteners or very little sugar and skim or low-fat milk in your tea or coffee. Most adults are aware that excess caffeine consumption can cause nervousness, irritability, anxiety, shakiness, insomnia, and an inability to relax and concentrate. It may also produce a temporary increase of heart rate and blood pressure and sometimes an irregular heartbeat in persons who are both hypertensive and normotensive. The content of caffeine is greater in coffee than in tea or soft drinks and least in cocoa and chocolate products. Therefore, it is best for most persons (particularly hypertensives) to consume no more than two cups of coffee,

four cups of tea, or four cans of caffeinated sodas (regular or diet sodas) daily. Chocolate should be limited (especially for young children). One benefit of drinking tea over other caffeinated or even decaffeinated beverages is that it contains antioxidants that are healthful. It is very helpful to read the labels on bottles or cans to determine the sugar and caloric content and whether it contains caffeine. Very few sweets or high-caloric snacks or drinks with lots of sugar should be available in the house.

7. Eating raw fruits or vegetables just before a meal or consuming a low-calorie soup with luncheon or dinner can be filling and can reduce hunger and the total calories consumed at a meal. It should be recalled that practically all soups, except gazpacho, have a high salt content.

8. It is important to remember that alcoholic drinks contain considerable amounts of carbohydrate calories without any nutritional value. **If alcohol is consumed, it is essential to avoid drinking more than one or two drinks per day,** not only to limit calories but also to prevent its effect on elevating blood pressure of individuals with hypertension.

9. It should be mentioned that when a person stops smoking, there will be a tendency to gain weight because the metabolic rate (the rate the body burns up calories in food) decreases when you stop smoking. This weight gain can be easily offset by an increase in physical activity—otherwise, it will require a further reduction in the food and calories consumed.

10. The use of a pedometer can be quite helpful in recording physical activity. It is recommended that 10,000 or more steps be taken each day to maintain adequate physical activity. The distance traveled depends, of course, on the stride of the individual, that is, the distance in feet made with each step (toe-to-toe or heel-to-heel). The average step taken by adults is about 2.5 feet; therefore,

10,000 steps per day by most adults is equivalent to about 4.73 miles. Charts that are supplied with your pedometer are available to convert stride length and steps taken to miles walked. Walking is very healthy and can be done by almost everyone, and it requires no special skills, equipment, or advanced conditioning. It is providential that over 2,000 years ago, Hippocrates, The Father of Medicine, said that "walking is man's best medicine." Obesity is relatively uncommon in societies throughout the world where individuals remain very active physically. Even in the United States, very few of the Amish, who are reported to be about six times as active as most Americans, become obese, despite a diet that is "heavy in meat, eggs, bread, and pies."

11. Currently, nine drugs are available that may help obese individuals lose weight. The most popular are orlistat (Xenical), which decreases digestion and absorption of some fats from the intestine. It inhibits about 30% of fat absorption; however, because it prevents absorption of some fat soluble vitamins (A, D, E, and beta-carotene), these must be replaced by taking vitamin pills 2 hours before or 2 hours after orlistat. It may cause some diarrhea, bloating, and abdominal pain. Sibutramine (Meridia) suppresses appetite and is modestly effective in causing weight loss; however, it may cause a slight increase in blood pressure and heart rate, nervousness, and insomnia. These drugs should be used only when prescribed by a physician.

12. Dieters should weigh themselves at least once a week and keep a record of their weight and also the food they eat each day. If at first you fail to lose weight, try again. With the proper diet, adequate exercise, and motivation, you CAN succeed!

13. Getting 7 to 9 hours of sleep daily appears to decrease the risk of obesity. It has recently been reported that persons sleeping only 6, 5, or 2–4 hours were 23%, 50%, and 73%, respectively, more likely to be obese than those getting 7 to 9 hours of sleep. A lack of sleep may increase the desire to eat and consume excess calories.

14. For those who are morbidly obese and unable to lose weight, surgical procedures to bypass the stomach should be considered. Morbid obesity refers to extremely obese individuals who are more than 100 pounds over their ideal healthy weight and have a BMI of greater than 40 (see **Table 2**). This may include 8% of American adults! Surgical procedures used to bypass the stomach decrease the amount of food absorbed and are known as bariatric surgery. Less food is eaten because patients experience a rapid sense of fullness even after eating a small meal. This surgery can cause marked weight loss that can be maintained, and it can be lifesaving. Furthermore, it is reported that about 80% of diabetics have their blood sugar return to normal levels after bypass procedures. However, the surgery can be very difficult, especially when obesity is very marked, and it has been reported that 1 of every 50 patients die from complications of these operations. Therefore, it is extremely important to have bariatric surgery performed at a medical center where surgeons have done a large number of these procedures and have developed special expertise. A variety of surgical procedures are now available; some reduce the stomach size and are reversible.

15. It is smart to shop for foods when you are *not* hungry because you will be less apt to buy additional items that are unnecessary and only add to calories you and your family might consume at home. It is also advisable to make a list of what you need and stick to it. You will also save money by buying less. Finally, it is recommended that you periodically shop for food with your children and make an effort to familiarize them about healthy foods and the importance of limiting fast foods and those that contain excess fat, sugar, and salt. Permitting children to aid you in making healthy choices can influence the food they consume and their future health. You can set a wonderful example that impacts you and your entire family.

RISKS *of Salt*

Table salt (sodium chloride) may play a role in contributing to high blood pressure in 50% to 60% of all people with hypertension. Table salt is composed of 40% sodium and 60% chloride, and it appears that the combination of both sodium *and* chloride is required to produce hypertension in laboratory animals and some humans. Decreasing salt in the diet and increased salt elimination caused by diuretics (water pills) can lower blood pressure in most people with hypertension. A strong relationship has been shown to exist between the amount of salt eaten and hypertension, and in certain experimental models, including apes, evidence indicates that excess salt consumption causes hypertension. Recent evidence indicates that excess salt consumption may cause damage to the heart and arteries of some people, even in the absence of hypertension.

In the hypertensive population, roughly 75% of Blacks and 50% of Whites are salt sensitive; that is, excess salt consumption will increase their blood pressure. Salt sensitivity is also common in individuals who are obese, individuals with diabetes, and persons older than 65 years. The only way to find out whether you are sensitive to salt is to see whether going from a low-salt to a high-salt diet increases your blood pressure or vice versa. The kidneys of salt-sensitive individuals do not eliminate excess dietary salt as well as the kidneys of normal persons. **Excess consumption of salt can cause water retention and constriction of arterioles (very small arteries) in salt-sensitive individuals, thereby increasing blood pressure; the reason for this arterial constriction remains unknown.**

Although the greater occurrence and greater severity of hypertension in Blacks than in Whites remain unexplained, it has been suggested that the kidneys of Blacks retain more salt. Some Blacks may consume less potassium than Whites which may explain why they have more severe hypertension; **potassium appears to oppose**

the accumulation of sodium in the body and can dilate arteries and decrease blood pressure.

Americans consume roughly 20 times the amount of sodium a person requires for normal body function. The Institute of Medicine reported that the body normally needs only about 180 mg of sodium each day to replace that eliminated in the urine, feces, and sweat. It is noteworthy that Yanomamie Indians, a primitive tribe in South America, eat only about 20 mg of sodium daily, and they remain healthy, do not gain weight with aging, and do not develop hypertension. On the other hand, 65 million Americans have hypertension (an increase of 30% since 1994), and with aging, about 90% will eventually develop hypertension! Dr. Claude Lenfant, former chairman of the National High Blood Pressure Education Program, recently stated that "damage to arteries begins at fairly low blood pressures—those formerly considered normal." Unfortunately, Americans have steadily increased their sodium consumption in the past 20 years, due mainly to increased food intake. A restaurant meal may contain more salt than should be consumed for the entire day. Furthermore, the average sodium content of food has increased about 6% in the past decade. **More than 75% of the sodium we eat comes from processed food (i.e., food prepared by companies for public consumption) and restaurant meals; about 12% comes from natural, unprocessed food, and about 11% is added in the household.** Persons with hypertension should read the labels on processed foods to become familiar with the amounts of sodium they are eating. **However, one must be aware that the sodium content indicated on the label is for *one* serving—individuals frequently eat more than a single serving. A daily dietary intake for adults of no more than 2,400 mg of sodium is recommended by health experts.** The average American now consumes about twice this amount. A reduction of sodium intake to 2,400 mg (about 1 teaspoonful of salt) daily appears both safe and achievable and can decrease the severity of hypertension. This restriction of sodium also might reduce the number of people developing hypertension each year by 20% and decrease the yearly mortality rate from stroke by 39% and heart attack by 30%. Reducing dietary sodium may increase the effectiveness of certain antihypertensive drugs and may eliminate the need for medication in some hypertensive persons. Individuals with hypertension would benefit most if they could limit their sodium consumption to no more than 1,500 mg daily. **It has been estimated that reducing the salt consumption of adult Americans by half would save 150,000 lives each year!** It has been said that salt "is perhaps the deadliest ingredient in the food supply." The less salt that is consumed the greater is the protection from the development of hypertension, stroke, heart, kidney, and arterial disease. Thus, don't take anything "with a grain of salt."

Limitation of processed and restaurant foods high in sodium, table salt, and salt used for cooking should be combined with other healthful lifestyle changes, such as weight reduction, smoking cessation, limited consumption of alcohol, adequate physical activity, and a diet that is low in saturated fat and cholesterol and high in fiber, fruits, and vegetables. Fresh foods contain very little sodium, and the addition of pepper, spices, herbs, lemon, onion, garlic, vinegar, table wine, horseradish, unsalted mustard, catsup (no added salt), and Worcestershire sauce (with low sodium) can add flavor to food and help break the salt habit. Be aware of the milligrams of sodium in your food, and use more foods that are labeled low sodium or unsalted. Keeping a record of your sodium consumption can be very helpful in achieving your goal to reduce dietary sodium. **Remember that the milligrams of sodium indicated on the label apply to one serving. If you consume two servings, you will, of course, be consuming twice the amount of sodium.**

Some common foods high in sodium are listed in **Table 7.** Other particularly high sources of sodium include tomato juice, Bloody

Mary mix, cocoa mix, canned soups, canned vegetables, bologna, smoked meats, bacon, frankfurters, ham, tuna packed in water or in oil, anchovies, sardines, pancake mix, salted potato chips, salted pretzels, salted popcorn, salted nuts, bread, waffles, butter, cheese, bouillon, catsup, dill pickles, sauerkraut, and baking powder/soda.

The Center for Science in the Public Interest (CSPI) reported the sodium content for 100 popular foods, and they found that different brands of similar foods often have wide variations in sodium content of 50% to 100% or more. It is noteworthy that the public usually cannot recognize these differences in sodium content. Differences reported in some popular foods with high sodium contents include: a small order of fries at Burger King has almost three times as much sodium as at McDonald's; Bumble Bee solid white Albacore tuna has more than twice as much sodium as Crown Prince's product; General Mills Honey Nut Cheerios has more than three times as much sodium as Barbara's Honey Nut O's; Safeway Premium Select BBQ Sauce contains about half as much sodium as Kraft BBQ Sauce; more sodium is present in small and medium hamburgers at Burger King than at McDonald's. Different brands of hot dogs, bacon, ham, sausage, breads, crackers, cheeses, pizzas, frozen foods, salad dressings, spaghetti sauces, salsa, potato and tortilla chips, chicken strips and nuggets, and soups often have significant differences in salt content. The sodium in almost all of these foods could be reduced without significantly altering flavor and decreasing acceptance by the public. Unfortunately, it is usually impossible to reduce sodium in soups without losing flavor; the one exception (as was pointed out to me by the late food critic, Craig Claiborne) is gazpacho soup, which depends largely on herbs and other seasoning for flavor rather than sodium.

Salt substitutes and "lite salt" should not be used without the recommendation of a physician. Many substitutes contain potassium, which may be hazardous to some—particularly those with impaired kidney function or those taking certain antihypertensive drugs that cause potassium retention. The use of salt tablets to counteract salt and water loss, even with excess sweating during physical activity and in hot weather, should be avoided unless recommended by a physician. However, individuals who sweat excessively may need to eat salty foods.

Individuals who are not highly conditioned and trained runners and who plan to run in a marathon should avoid consuming large amounts of water (e.g., 13 cups, or more than 100 ounces) during the race. Studies indicate that slow runners are particularly apt to stop frequently to drink excess water. This can substantially lower the sodium concentration in the blood to critical levels, which can cause acute illness with confusion, nausea, and rarely seizures, coma, and death.

Marathon running is a relatively safe sport; however, the belief that you should "stay ahead of your thirst" has been replaced by "drink when you are thirsty." Low salt concentrations in the blood can be avoided if excess water consumption is avoided. Sports drinks are not protective, as they supply more water than salt. Adequate water consumption during exercise, military operations, and desert hikes, especially in hot weather, is vital to prevent illness from heat and dehydration and to maintain performance. However, it is safest to drink only when you are thirsty.

For individuals who are particularly fond of salt, limiting salt eventually will decrease the desire for this compound. In a brief period, food begins to taste better without it. **Use less salt and more herbs and spices when preparing food. Purchase foods that are low in salt and ask for foods that are low in salt when eating out.**

The need to reduce salt consumption in the United States should be a top priority because excess salt very significantly contributes to the development of hypertension and its compli-

Table 7 Examples of Common Foods with Sodium Levels		
Food	Amount	Sodium (mg)
Canned bouillon	1 cup	782
Canned juice, tomato	½ cup	438
Canned meat	1 oz	394
Canned soup, chicken noodle	1 cup	849
Canned soup, lentil with ham	1 cup	1,319
Canned spaghetti and meatballs	1 cup	940
Cheese:		
Cream	1 oz	84
Swiss	1 oz	73
American, processed	1 oz	405
Low-sodium cheddar or colby	1 oz	6
Frankfurter, beef	1 serving	461
Canned olives	3	120
Pickles, dill	1 spear	384
Pizza, cheese	1 slice	336
Pot pie, beef	1 serving	736
Pot pie, turkey	1 serving	1,390
Salad dressing, Thousand Island	1 tpsp	109
Italian sausage	1 link	665
Soy sauce	1 tbsp	1,005
Frozen dinner, fried chicken with mashed potatoes and corn	1 serving	1,500
Frozen dinner, meat loaf with mashed potatoes and carrots	1 serving	1,943

Source: U.S. Department of Agriculture, Agriculture Research Service. USDA nutrient database for standard reference. Nutrient Data Laboratory home page, http://www.nal.usda.gov/fnic/foodcomp

cations of brain, heart, kidney, and blood vessel disease. Unfortunately, the public pays insufficient attention to limiting dietary salt but are much more concerned with the fats, carbohydrates, and calories they consume. Furthermore, none of the currently popular diets mention the importance of reducing salt consumption. Only the DASH diet emphasizes the importance and benefit of dietary salt reduction, especially in persons with hypertension.

The fact that salt plays such a significant role in both the development and severity of hypertension and its complications mandates that greater efforts be made to decrease its use. Increased efforts are needed to:

1. Inform hypertensive patients and the public about the risks of using excess salt
2. Indicate the salt content of foods consumed in restaurants
3. Eliminate products containing lots of salt, fats, and sugar from school menus and dispensing machines
4. Curtail marketing of foods with high salt content

These efforts may be helpful. However, as the National High Blood Pressure Education Program and the Center for Science in the Public Interest have repeatedly indicated, the only really successful way of decreasing salt consumption is to reduce the salt content of processed foods and to introduce new palatable foods with much less salt that will be accepted by the public.

Physical Activity and Exercise—RISKS of Inactivity

Exercise is essential for health and physical fitness. Unfortunately, Americans have recently tended to be passive spectators rather than active participants in physical activities, exercise, and sports. About 40% of adults do not engage in any leisure-time physical activity. Furthermore, our children and teenagers have become obsessed with television and computers. Computer games are especially popular. **It is reported that about 25% of children in America spend 4 or more hours per day watching television and that many spend 7 hours a day in front of a television or computer screen!** Surprisingly, children 3 years old or less watch television between 2 and 3 hours daily. During these years, the brain of a child is rapidly undergoing nerve growth and developing connections; although not proven, recent evidence suggests that excess exposure to television at this young age may influence brain development and result in difficulty concentrating (attention deficit) during school years and later. **It is strongly recommended that children 2 years old or less do not watch television.**

A study of 10-year-old American girls revealed a direct correlation between hours spent watching TV and excess body fat. A survey in one city revealed that 60% of children had a TV in their room, and they were three times more likely to be overweight than those without TVs. **The American Academy of Pediatrics recommends limiting TV and video viewing to no more than 2 hours daily.** Eating high-caloric foods and drinking sodas and other beverages full of sugar while watching TV and consuming lots of buttered popcorn, nachos, candy, and other high-caloric foods and sodas at the movies or sporting events can contribute significantly to weight gain and obesity.

The increasing time spent in front of computers will further erode participation in physical activity and reduce physical fitness. Only 27% of high school students engage in moderate physical activity for at least 30 minutes daily for 5 or more days each week. Only 22% of adults exercise for at least 30 minutes during most days. **Up** to 80% of Americans do not exercise regularly, and 40% do not exercise at all.

Of great concern is that three out of four children who are overweight or obese at the ages of 9 to 13 years will remain so when adults. It appears that inadequate physical activity, especially common among individuals with lower levels of education and income, is a major contributor to obesity. Surprisingly, recent studies have found that many living in the suburbs are more obese than those living in cities. Apparently, suburbanites constantly use cars for transportation because stores and shopping centers are often miles away from their homes. Furthermore, sidewalks are frequently not available in the suburbs, and suburbanites walk much less than city dwellers. Physical inactivity exerts a particularly strong influence in the development of obesity in children.

There has been an unfortunate trend for public schools in the United States to decrease or eliminate PE (physical education) in the belief that using the time for academic instruction is preferable. This is a very serious mistake that must be reversed. After-school programs are extremely important for the health and welfare of our children. The period from 3 to 6 PM is when most children and teenagers get into trouble by smoking, using drugs and alcohol, committing crimes, and becoming involved in fights or serious gang wars. Responsible supervision during this critical period is crucial. **Physical exercise is important not only for physical health, but also for mental health because it can reduce emotional tension and provide a sense of well-being.**

One of my patients was under considerable stress as an executive in his company. He reported that at the end of each workday he returned home and would walk into the woods nearby and scream for prolonged periods. This was his way of releasing anxiety and frustration. He said he had no time for exercise or relaxation, and he hardly ever took a lunch break. When I discovered that he had been a track star in college, I urged him to find time to jog regularly. Subsequently, he confided that jogging regularly had an enormous beneficial effect on his life and on his relationship with his family and associates.

Parents, schools, and the government should demand regular physical exercise periods for all students. Finally, **it is especially valuable if parents can participate with their children in extracurricular and community physical activity and sporting events. This will help children develop and enjoy regular exercise.**

Schools often emphasize team sports and the importance of winning. As a consequence, some children and teenagers with limited athletic ability who would love to participate in sports are left idle on the sidelines with little or no exercise and with poor self-esteem and a sense of inferiority. Such inactivity must not be permitted; **every child and teenager should be involved regularly in a sports program. Encouragement can do wonders for children and teenagers: "none should be left behind."**

Sedentary persons ("couch potatoes") are more likely to be overweight or obese and eventually to develop hypertension, heart attacks, strokes, diabetes, and elevated harmful fats in the blood than those who are physically active. Regular, moderate aerobic exercise (i.e., dynamic exercise that increases oxygen intake and increases activity of the heart, lungs, and muscles) can reduce systolic blood pressure (the higher pressure in the arteries when the heart is contracting) and diastolic blood pressure (the lower pressure in the arteries when the heart is not contracting) by about 10 and 8 mm Hg (mercury), respectively, in hypertensive subjects. **Moderate-intensity training appears to be just as effective as, if not better than, high-intensity exercise in providing many beneficial effects.** To keep most physically fit, it is preferable that various exercises be used periodically so that all the major muscles will be strengthened.

The benefits of regularly performing moderate aerobic exercise are many:

- Proper weight is maintained more easily.
- Muscle mass, strength, and agility are increased and preserved.
- The risks of osteoporosis and diabetes are diminished. Weight bearing, for example, walking, running, jogging, and weight lifting, is important in protecting against osteoporosis. (Swimming, although an excellent muscle exercise, is not weight bearing and is not protective against osteoporosis; it is noteworthy that the weightlessness occurring in space flights causes astronauts to lose considerable amounts of calcium in their urine.)
- Elevated blood pressure may be reduced.
- Damage to the coronary arteries of the heart may be prevented and heart function improved, and the chance of a heart attack is decreased in both men and women.
- Levels of the "good" blood cholesterol (HDL), which protects against hardening of the arteries, may be increased, whereas levels of the "bad" cholesterol (LDL) and triglycerides (blood fats) usually decrease.
- Emotional tension, anxiety, anger, and depression may be significantly alleviated; the chance of heart attack and sudden death caused by excessive emotional or physical stress may be reduced.
- The occurrence of colon and breast cancer may be decreased.
- Inflammation and pain may be reduced in the joints of patients with some types of arthritis.
- Mental decline in older persons may be delayed.

Researchers have shown that exercise benefits the heart by improving the ability of the heart arteries to dilate in response to a substance (nitric oxide) released from the lining of these arteries. This dilation occurs even in the presence of atherosclerosis (hardening of the arteries). Also, most recently, it has been reported that "regular moderate exercise not only increases muscle use of energy, but also enhances formation of new nerve cells in areas of the brain that support memory."

Exercise intensity and duration for adults should be increased gradually and then performed for 30 or more minutes 5 or preferably all days of the week. For children, 60 minutes of moderate physical activity most (preferably all) days of the week is recommended. Individuals older than 40 years or anyone with any indication of heart or vascular disease should consult a physician before embarking on an exercise program. A variety of stress tests can provide valuable information about the coronary arteries and function of your heart and the degree to which you can safely exercise. Furthermore, your physician probably will want to check your blood levels of sugar and cholesterol and sometimes may determine levels of homocysteine and c-reactive protein (CRP) chemicals that may be involved in hardening of the arteries. Any elevations of these chemicals may require medication with drugs, such as the statins, which can lower elevated levels of the bad cholesterol and CRP, and folic acid, which can lower homocysteine.

It is especially important to choose enjoyable activities and exercises—if they are boring, they will not be continued for very long. Walking and jogging are particularly popular types of exercise that can be performed alone, with a few friends, or in large groups. Bicycling, basketball, soccer, tennis, paddle tennis, squash, volleyball, cross-country skiing, skating, roller-blading, golf, swimming, aerobic group exercise, or dancing are excellent ways of getting the exercise needed to improve cardiovascular fitness and muscle strength. Even regularly performed light-intensity exercise, such as Tai Chi, may reduce blood pressure modestly.

Exercise machines (such as the treadmill, stationary bicycle, rowing machine, stair climber, and the vast array of dynamic muscle-building machines) are excellent and very convenient ways to work out; the opportunity to watch television, listen to music, or even read while using these machines can make the physical activity more enjoyable. Most of these moderate-intensity exercises pose little chance of injury, especially if a few minutes of muscle stretching—a warm-up period—precede the exercise. Stretching after exercise is also beneficial in preventing muscle soreness and stiffness.

One word of caution regarding the use of a Walkman if walking or jogging on a road: the possibility of being hit by a car is increased if hearing is impaired. Jogging or walking is safer if done against traffic so that you can see and avoid oncoming vehicles.

Although exercise will briefly increase systolic pressure, systolic and diastolic pressures may be lower for as long as several hours after the activity ends. No evidence suggests that regular, moderate-intensity exercise increases the risk of stroke or heart attack in hypertensive individuals who have no heart disease or previous history of vascular disease of the brain. However, exercise may have to be limited for those with heart disease or other disabling conditions; if hypertension is severe, it should be controlled with antihypertensive medication before embarking on an exercise program.

Lifting or "pressing" very heavy weights will build skeletal muscles; however, the straining required with this exercise, known as isometrics (requiring extreme muscle contraction), definitely should be avoided, especially if you have hypertension. This type of activity can elevate both systolic and diastolic pressures, with systolic pressures sometimes reaching 300 mm Hg or higher! Severe elevations of blood pressure could be especially hazardous for anyone using aspirin or anticoagulants. Repetitive light weight lifting or exercises requiring intermittent contraction and relaxation of muscles, if not strenuous, are permissible.

Moderately intense exercise for 30 minutes will burn up approximately 150 calories. If it is more desirable to perform two 15-minute or three 10-minute periods of exercise, the benefit and the total calories burned will be similar. Men burn up 10% to 20% more calories than women during exercise, probably because of men's larger muscle mass. The number of calories burned up also depends on a person's weight, the type and intensity of exercise, and the time spent exercising. For example, in 1 hour, a person weighing 150 pounds would burn up about 325 calories walking 4 mph, whereas bicycling 15 mph or running at a pace of 1 mile every 10 minutes would burn up about 720 calories. **Table 8** reveals the approximate number of calories a 150-pound person would burn up in 1 hour performing various physical activities. (A heavier person would burn up more calories than a lighter person performing the same amount of exercise.)

Physical activity, when combined with a reduced caloric intake, can significantly lower weight and thereby further reduce blood pressure.

A good measure of fitness is your heart rate and length of time you can continue on a treadmill at different degrees of exercise. The maximum heart rate (pulse) you can achieve during exercise decreases with age. The pulse rate at your wrist caused by exercising should be recorded (measure beats for 6 seconds immediately after exercise and multiply by 10 to calculate the beats per minute). With moderate exercise, this number in the normal, healthy individual should be roughly equivalent to 220 minus your age (the formula for maximum rate) multiplied by 70% (the recommended percent of the maximum rate that should be attained during moderate exercise). Certain drugs (e.g., beta blockers used to treat hypertension) may slow the heart-rate response to exercise. Any

Table 8 Average Calories Burned in 30 Minutes by a Person Weighing 150 Pounds During Physical Activity.			

(Persons weighing less burn less, and persons weighing more burn more calories in 30 minutes)

Aerobic dancing (low impact)	172	Ping Pong	135
Badminton	225	Raking	112
Basketball (game)	330	Raquetball	308
Basketball (leisurely, non-game)	195	Rowing (leisurely)	112
Bicycling, 10 mph (6 minutes/mile)	188	Rowing machine	270
Bicycling, 13 mph (4.6 minutes/mile)	300	Running, 08 mph (7.5 minutes/mile)	458
Billiard	68	Running, 09 mph (6.7 minutes/mile)	495
Bowling	82	Running, 10 mph (6 minutes/mile)	525
Canoeing, 2.5 mph	105	Scuba diving	285
Canoeing, 4.0 mph	202	Shopping for groceries	90
Croquet	90	Skipping rope	428
Cross country snow skiing, intense	495	Snow shoveling	292
Cross country snow skiing, leisurely	232	Snow skiing, downhill	195
Cross country snow skiing, moderate	330	Soccer	292
Dancing (slow)	82	Squash	308
Gardening, moderate	135	Stair climbing	210
Golfing (walking, w/o cart)	150	Swimming (25 yards/minute)	180
Golfing (with a cart)	105	Swimming (50 yards/minute)	338
Handball	345	Tennis	240
Hiking with a 10 lb. load	270	Tennis (doubles)	165
Hiking with a 20 lb. load	300	Vacuuming	112
Hiking with a 30 lb. load	352	Volleyball (game)	180
Hiking, no load	232	Volleyball (leisurely)	105
Ironing	75	Walking, 2 mph (30 minutes/mile)	90
Jogging, 5 mph (12 minutes/mile)	278	Walking, 3 mph (20 minutes/mile)	120
Jogging, 6 mph (10 minutes/mile)	345	Walking, 4 mph (15 minutes/mile)	150
Mowing	202	Waterskiing	240

Source: http://www.nutribase.com/exercala.htm

abnormalities of heart response to exercise should be reported to a physician.

Most antihypertensive medications do not interfere with the ability to exercise. Some drugs (beta blockers) that partially block the response of the heart to exercise, however, will limit the pumping action of the heart and slow the pulse. Consequently, these drugs may reduce a person's capacity for strenuous physical activity.

From this discussion, it should be obvious that the adage "no pain, no gain" does not apply to exercise. Regularly performed, moderately intense, nonpainful exercise can be both enjoyable and beneficial to health. **Strenuous exercise is not required or recommended to lose weight and stay fit.** Thus, if there are no medical reasons to avoid or limit physical activity, start exercising regularly and discover the many ways to enjoy it!

RISKS of Alcohol

Alcohol is consumed at social gatherings and with meals by many adults throughout most of the world. Even children are permitted a modest amount of wine with meals in some countries. **Small amounts of alcohol can be part of a healthy diet, and it is estimated that 50% to 75% of American adults drink alcohol.** In the United States, it is illegal to sell or serve alcohol to persons under the age of 21 years; however, the use of alcohol by individuals in their teens and at college is extremely common.

Alcohol has become the drug of choice among adolescents (teenagers). Three of four teenagers have tried alcohol. **Also, more than one in three senior high school students and about half of 21 year olds are occasionally heavy (binge) drinkers (binge drinking is defined as consuming five or more drinks in a row for males and four or more for females).** A new dangerous challenge practiced by some is to drink 21 alcoholic beverages upon turning 21 years old within a period of 2 to 3 hours, before the facility serving the alcohol closes. Tragically, a number of deaths have resulted from this senseless practice. Especially disturbing is a trend to drink earlier and more frequently and to consume more alcohol. **It is estimated that 20% to 30% of teenagers who drink frequently are potential or established chronic alcoholics (those addicted to alcohol)! Parents must remain alert to recognize any evidence that their children are drinking alcohol. With signs of alcohol abuse (e.g., breath smelling of alcohol, unsteady drunken behavior with slurred speech, drunk-driving arrests, frequent arguments, secretive behavior, and a lack of interest in school work and athletics), parents must intervene and sometimes seek professional help.** The younger the age when a child starts to drink alcohol, the greater the chance of becoming a problem drinker. **It is important that alcohol not be accessible to children in the home.**

It is a startling fact that the leading cause of death in teenagers results from reckless driving while intoxicated. Recently, the death rate from car crashes has decreased significantly in the United States, partly the result of more difficult requirements and testing for obtaining a driver's license. Most college students admit to driving while drunk or being driven by someone who has been drinking. Alcohol intoxication distorts judgment, impairs coordination, and delays reflexes, which explains the extreme danger of driving a car or operating any potentially dangerous equipment that requires dexterity, judgment, and concentration. In the United States in the year 2000, there were nearly two alcohol-related traffic deaths per hour, 43 per day, and 303 per week. A person with a blood alcohol level of 0.08 mg % or more is legally considered intoxicated; however, a level of even 0.02 mg % (which can result from just 1 drink) may impair driving ability! Therefore, it is safest to avoid any alcohol if you are going to drive a vehicle.

Chronic alcoholism can cause serious liver, brain, heart, and nerve damage and can destroy an individual's relationship with family and friends. It also will disrupt the individual's ability to perform a job successfully. It is reported that approximately 85,000 deaths yearly in the United States result from alcohol-related injuries or disease. It is the third most common cause of preventable deaths; only smoking or obesity cause more preventable deaths.

Case Report

H.L. was an extremely attractive and likable young gentleman who was always great fun to be with because he had a delightful sense of humor and was knowledgeable on all the latest stories and social gossip. He was always the life of the party. Unfortunately, this popularity played a significant role in his excessive consumption of alcohol with his many friends.

By the time he was 30 years old, he was a chronic alcoholic. He would regularly have several drinks at lunch, and then he always would consume additional alcohol in the late afternoon and during and after dinner. As a result, he was unable to function effectively in any capacity. He lost his job, and his role as a husband and father of two children progressively deteriorated. Drinking seemed to help him temporarily escape from his problems and depression, and he became addicted to alcohol.

When he was 40 years old, he developed jaundice (a yellowish color of his skin and eyes). Medical examination and tests revealed that he had developed cirrhosis (a scarring) of the liver with accumulation of fluid in his abdomen and swelling of his ankles. Although the doctor explained the seriousness of his condition, he chose to continue drinking and would not eat regularly.

When he was 43 years old, dilated veins in his swallowing tube (esophageal varices) were discovered. These varices resulted from cirrhosis of his liver, and the doctor discussed with him the potentially deadly nature of this condition. For the first time, H.L. seemed to grasp the seriousness of his condition, and with the help of medication and the guidance of his doctor, he was able to stop drinking alcohol. He also began attending AA (Alcoholics Anonymous) meetings and began eating a healthy diet. He felt remarkably improved physically and mentally, and his relationship with his wife and children began to normalize. The renewed happiness in his family was touching to behold. He was now once again playing first-rate golf, which he loved. Despite this new lease on life, he experienced a massive hemorrhage from a rupture of his esophageal varices. Efforts to stop the bleeding and repeated transfusions were ineffective, and he died within 1 hour after the bleeding started. This story is not uncommon in chronic alcoholics who develop cirrhosis. The tragedy is that this gentleman made every effort to stop drinking and rebuild his life, yet the damage to his liver was irreversible because of prolonged alcohol abuse. **Figure 8** indicates the serious consequences of excessive consumption of alcohol.

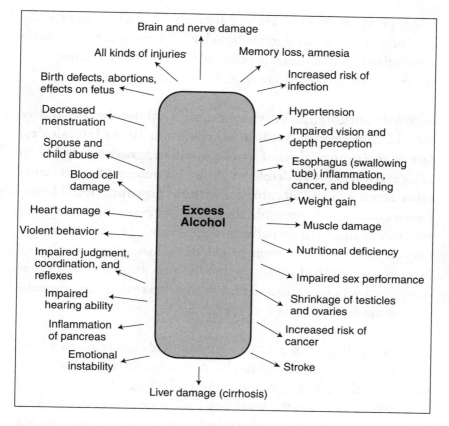

Figure 8 Conditions often occurring with excess alcohol consumption.

Perhaps 7% to 10% of all cases of hypertension in the United States are caused by excess alcohol consumption; even consumption of only four drinks daily may elevate blood pressure. Men with hypertension who consume alcohol should limit their intake to no more than two drinks of spirits (1.5 ounces of 80% proof), two 12-ounce cans of beer, or two 4- to 5- ounce glasses of wine each day. Women, small men, those over the age of 65 years, and those who are frail should limit their intake to half this amount. Such modest alcohol consumption rarely elevates

89

blood pressure. Modest alcohol intake may slightly elevate the level of good cholesterol in the blood, which protects arteries from accumulating cholesterol deposits and may decrease the occurrence of heart attacks, as compared with that of teetotalers.

Alcohol consumption provides a significant number of calories (one 12-ounce can or bottle of beer contains 100 to 150 calories; one 4- to 5-ounce glass of wine contains approximately 125 to 150 calories, and two drinks or about 1.5 ounces of spirits contains about 125 to 150 calories) without any nutritional benefit—a point worth remembering! Alcohol consumption should certainly be limited in hypertensive individuals. If you have hypertension and find that even moderate consumption of alcohol increases your blood pressure, then do not drink alcohol! Consumption by an individual of four to five drinks daily usually indicates some dependence on alcohol.

Evidence gathered in France suggests that consumption of red wine may offer protection from heart attacks. Although the explanation for this effect remains unclear, phenolic chemicals in red wine, which decrease the tendency for arteries to harden and for blood clots to form, may play a role. However, excess consumption of wine in France accounts for the highest prevalence of cirrhosis (liver damage) in the world. There is also evidence that daily consumption of a small amount of red wine may reduce the risk of prostate cancer—perhaps because of the presence of an antioxidant.

If a heavy drinker wishes to curtail his or her alcohol consumption, this reduction should occur gradually. Abrupt cessation of alcohol intake can stimulate the sympathetic nervous system and liberate hormones (adrenaline and noradrenaline), which then can constrict arteries and sometimes cause severe hypertension. Heavy drinkers should consult a physician and develop a program for cessation of drinking so as to minimize or prevent

symptoms of alcohol withdrawal (delirium tremens, i.e., DTs) such as anxiety, shakiness, insomnia, increased pulse, temperature, and respiration, upset stomach, and sometimes confusion, hallucinations (objects and people appear abnormal and distorted), and convulsions (seizures).

A prolonged period of rehabilitation may be necessary, and permanent abstinence from alcohol is essential. Often, regularly attending AA meetings may be very helpful and provide the necessary support for reformed alcoholics to remain sober. **They should never drink any kind of alcohol at any time in the future because even *one drink* may cause them to revert to chronic alcoholism.**

Finally, alcohol consumption may enhance the effects of some antihypertensive and sedative medications and illicit drugs, leading to a decrease in blood pressure or oversedation that may cause one to feel faint and unsteady or fall asleep. These interactions can be particularly hazardous while driving a car.

RISKS *of Cigarette Smoking*

There is no more treacherous contributor to health problems than cigarette smoking. Even smoke from cigars or pipes is hazardous to health. The havoc smoking causes is monumental, and it is the most preventable cause of premature death in the United States. Despite strong antismoking campaigns indicating the serious health risks of smoking, in 2002, 46 million adults in the United States smoked (i.e., about 22% of the adult population). Smoking causes more than 1,190 deaths per day and 20% of all deaths, and smoking-related medical care costs approximately $157 billion annually. In addition, up to 15% of daily smokers develop lung cancer, which causes no symptoms when it first develops, and after diagnosis, only about 15% of patients survive 5 years. **Smoking causes more deaths from cancer than deaths from breast, colon, and prostate cancer combined.** The conditions frequently resulting from cigarette smoking are shown in **Figure 9.**

Smoking accounts for several alarming statistics:

- 30% of cardiovascular deaths (including heart attack, heart failure, stroke, and blood vessel damage)
- 30% of all cancer deaths (including 87% of lung cancer deaths)
- 80% of deaths from chronic obstructive lung disease (primarily emphysema)

Consider this sobering fact: smoking cigarettes causes cancer of the lung and of the larynx (the "voice box"), chronic bronchitis, coronary heart disease, hardening of the arteries (atherosclerosis), cancer of the mouth and of the esophagus (the tube from the mouth to the stomach), chronic obstructive lung disease, low birth weight babies, unsuccessful pregnancies, increased infant mortality, and peptic ulcer. Although unproven, smoking may contribute to the development of cancer of the urinary bladder, pancreas, kidneys, and stomach. In addition, smoking appears

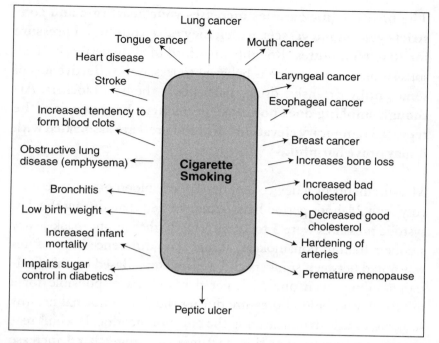

Figure 9 Conditions that may occur with cigarette smoking.

to be associated with stroke and possibly cataracts, bowel disease, macular degeneration (which impairs or destroys vision), and breast cancer. It can decrease the good cholesterol (HDL) and increase the bad cholesterol (LDL) in the blood. It also may cause platelets (small blood cells) to form clots that can block circulation and cause a heart attack or stroke. **Smoking results in a greater tendency to form blood clots in girls and women who are taking birth control pills.**

Smoking a pipe or cigars may be less injurious to a person's health than inhaling cigarette smoke. **Nevertheless, any form of smoking still poses a significant risk not only to the smoker, but also to all those who inhale the smoke passively ("second-hand smoke").**

The nicotine in cigarettes increases your heart rate and constricts your blood vessels, which may raise your blood pressure for 30 to 60 minutes. Roughly one third of all hypertensive persons smoke, and nicotine is believed to lessen the effectiveness of some antihypertensive drugs, particularly the beta blockers. **Although smoking does not cause permanent hypertension, the repeated temporary elevations of blood pressure associated with it may prove harmful.**

Measurements by a device that determines blood pressure repeatedly for a 24-hour period have demonstrated that, during the day, systolic pressures were 5 to 10 mm Hg higher in one-pack-a-day smokers than in nonsmokers; at night, no difference in pressures was noted between smokers and nonsmokers. Based on this finding, smoking even one pack per day appears responsible for a mildly elevated blood pressure during the day in normal healthy subjects, clearly demonstrating the effect of nicotine. It seems reasonable to suggest that this daytime, smoking-related increase would augment the blood pressure of hypertensive individuals and possibly increase the risk of complications.

Nicotine activates the sympathetic nervous system and thereby releases hormones (adrenaline and noradrenaline) into the circulation that not only increase your heart rate and blood pressure, but also may cause irregular heartbeats. In addition, **smoking decreases the supply of oxygen to tissues and vital organs. It adds carbon monoxide to the blood, which may damage blood vessels, permit cholesterol accumulation in the arteries, and accelerate hardening of the arteries. Indeed, the arteries of the heart (coronary arteries) are damaged more frequently and more severely in smokers than in nonsmokers.**

Although heavy or chain smokers are at greater risk than light smokers for developing the diseases mentioned previously, **non-smokers exposed to cigarette smoke from others ("passive smo-**

king") also are at increased risk for heart and lung disease. Indeed, persons living with a cigarette smoker have a 30% greater chance of developing heart disease than if they were not exposed to smoke. Such passive smoking is estimated to cause 37,000 deaths yearly. **Children of parents who smoke are also more likely to suffer from lung infections and asthma than children not exposed to smoke.**

Cigarette smokers without any obvious health problems are two to three times more likely to have a heart attack than nonsmokers, and the chances of surviving a heart attack usually are worse for smokers. The presence of high blood pressure, elevated blood cholesterol, diabetes, or obesity in smokers all further increases the risk of heart attack, stroke, and blood vessel damage (hardening of the arteries with a blockage or rupture of these vessels). **Smokers with hypertension are three to five times more likely to die from a heart attack or heart failure than nonsmokers and twice as likely to die of a stroke.** As the number of risk factors increases, so does the risk of premature death; with each additional risk factor, the chance of death may double. If all risk factors are present, the chance of premature death is enormous.

Despite these facts, 50 million Americans continue to smoke. Sadly, the number of teenage smokers is increasing, especially young women. Of considerable concern is that children and teenagers can easily purchase cigarettes through the Internet without having to establish that they are legally old enough (18 years or older) to do so. **Three thousand teenagers and children (many under 9 years of age) begin smoking each day!** It is estimated that one third of high school seniors are cigarette smokers. Also, the number of college students who smoke has increased by about 28% in the past few years. Psychosocial (i.e., emotional and social experiences) and peer pressures play a central role in influencing attitudes of many teenagers. Unfortunately, tobacco advertisements and the portrayal of smoking in movies glamorize cigarette smoking. Some young women apparently smoke to stay slim, as smoking increases body metabolism and burns more calories and also can curb the appetite. Ironically, one young man who was employed as a robust cowboy model to advertise a popular brand of cigarettes died of lung cancer because of smoking.

Recent evidence indicates that the younger a person is when starting to smoke, the greater the chance of cell damage and development of lung cancer. **Parents and teachers must present information to children at an early age about the very serious risks of smoking and should make every possible effort to prevent children from smoking. Because nicotine is an extremely addictive chemical, prevention is more effective than efforts to persuade a smoker to stop. Teenagers who do not smoke cigarettes are less likely to use illicit drugs.**

It has been reported that 90% of individuals who are chronic alcoholics also smoke cigarettes; evidence suggests that chronic excess alcohol consumption may increase the pleasure derived from smoking. Alcoholism appears to occur much more commonly in smokers than nonsmokers.

The good news is that 40 million Americans have given up smoking. Additional good news is that 1 year after cessation of smoking, the risk of cardiovascular disease diminishes markedly. The risk of heart disease decreases by approximately 50%, and at 5 years after smoking cessation, the risk of heart disease is almost the same as with nonsmokers. The risks of lung and other cancers, strokes, and chronic lung disease decrease as well. After 10 to 15 years of not smoking, the chances of death from a smoking-related disease are nearly as low as those of persons who never smoked.

Cessation of cigarette smoking is the most effective and important life insurance policy available. For your sake and for the

health of your family and all of those with whom you come in contact, *give it up***!**

Finally, "smokeless tobacco" should also be mentioned as harmful. There are two types: snuff and chewing tobacco. Snuff may be inhaled through the nose or placed between the cheek and gum. A wad of chewing tobacco also can be placed between the cheek and gum. Tobacco use in this manner may cause not only nicotine addiction, but also cancer of the mouth, tongue, larynx, and esophagus. In addition, such tobacco use can cause gum recession and tooth disease and increase the risk of heart disease. The addiction may be so severe in some individuals that they choose to sleep with a wad of tobacco between their gum and cheek so that nicotine is constantly absorbed into their body.

Many athletes, especially baseball players, chew and spit tobacco; about 92% of smokeless tobacco users are males, and about 2% are adolescents (ages 12 to 17 years). In the past few years the popularity of smokeless tobacco has increased among young adults and children. **Regrettably, adolescents view smokeless tobacco as a safe alternative to cigarettes, which, of course, is false.** Furthermore, adolescents who chew tobacco are much more likely to become cigarette smokers. The serious health risks of smokeless tobacco are very compelling reasons to stop tobacco chewing. Cancer of the mouth is one serious complication that occurs even in the relatively young. The method of quitting this habit is similar to that recommended for cigarette smokers.

Case Report

I.S. had smoked cigarettes since she was in her teens. She was a highly intelligent individual who appreciated the risks of smoking, yet she chose to continue. When 75 years old, she developed a hoarseness in her voice. She was seen at the Mayo Clinic in

Scottsdale, Arizona, where her left vocal cord was found to be paralyzed, and a tumor mass was discovered in the upper left lobe of her lung.

She was referred to the Mayo Clinic in Rochester, Minnesota, for surgical removal of the tumor. However, the extent of the tumor made removal impossible. She was subsequently given intensive radiation to the head and to the chest region overlying the tumor. In addition, she received repeated treatments of chemotherapy. Gradually, the tumor disappeared, and her voice returned to normal. About 95% of lung cancers are fatal within a few years. Although I.S. lived for 7 more years, the treatments she received caused her considerable weakness and disability accompanied by several falls and hip fractures, which significantly impaired the quality of her life. In the end, she elected to suspend all further treatment. Her courage and composure and her concern for others rather than herself inspired all who knew her. Although the tumor responded remarkably to treatment, side effects of repeated intensive chemotherapy and radiation were devastating, leaving her without the will to live.

Case Report

D.J. had smoked cigarettes since he was a teenager. It was the "cool" thing to do when he was growing up. The deadly consequences of smoking were not appreciated when he started smoking. He and so many of his friends became addicted to the nicotine in cigarettes, and many became heavy smokers (2 to 3 packs per day). Some became chain smokers.

In his early 60s, D.J. began to experience increasing shortness of breath with even mild exertion. After consulting with his physician, he was referred to a lung specialist. A series of tests revealed that his lungs had been severely damaged by heavy cigarette smoking over many years and that his lungs were unable to remove oxygen effectively from the air he breathed in and transport it to his blood. The oxygen content of his blood was markedly below normal and inadequate for his body to function normally; consequently, he became progressively more short of breath.

Eventually, it was necessary for him to carry an oxygen tank wherever he went in order to prevent him from gasping for air. The damage to his quality of life was devastating. This crippling and dreaded lung disease is called emphysema. Generally, little can be done, and usually the disease is progressive. D.J. died in his late 60s.

How to Quit Smoking

With any form of addiction, whether alcohol, drugs, or cigarette smoking, motivation is absolutely essential in quitting. Without sufficient commitment to abstain, the smoking cessation plan has little, if any, chance of success. **To underscore the importance of motivation, note that 95% of the 40 million persons who have quit smoking have done it on their own.** The poor success rates of many formal smoking cessation programs are most likely related to insufficient MOTIVATION.

To quit smoking is extremely difficult, especially for the heavy smoker, because most smokers are physically and psychologically addicted. However, the fear of disease caused by cigarette smoking has affected Americans very significantly, and tobacco consumption has decreased by 25% during the past 20 years. Today, physicians in this country rarely smoke because they are acutely aware of the enormous health risks. Unfortunately, the seriousness of the health hazards of smoking has not been sufficiently transmitted to populations outside of the United States; in most other countries, smoking remains prevalent at all levels of society and in all professions.

Millions of Americans try to give up smoking each year, but only 10% are successful on the first attempt. Persistence plus firm motivation are keys to success. Nearly two thirds of all those who repeatedly try to quit eventually succeed. Also, it is never too late to quit, given that health benefits may be gained by abstaining from this habit, no matter what the age of the individual and how long the duration of cigarette smoking.

There is no magic formula for smoking cessation. Some smokers respond to one approach better than another. Although smoking is physically addictive because of nicotine, it also results in strong psychologic and social dependence because it becomes associated with a large variety of situations and emotional states. Stressful situations may be lessened and concentration improved by smoking, which makes it especially desirable under some circumstances.

Repeatedly smoking at a particular time of the day, under a large variety of emotionally stressful circumstances, and during special social events and periods of entertainment can ingrain the habit and trigger the desire to smoke automatically at these times. For smoking cessation to be most successful, certain steps should be followed.

First and foremost, an earnest desire to quit smoking is essential. **You should be prepared to experience short-term discomfort (irritability, anxiety, and loss of concentration), which becomes most noticeable 2 to 4 days after cessation but usually disappears within 10 to 14 days.** Thereafter, the desire to smoke may occur periodically for months or years later, but this urge usually lasts only a few seconds. **It is extremely important to appreciate that anyone who has been a heavy smoker cannot become a "social smoker." Any "slip"—even smoking one cigarette—will very likely cause full resumption of smoking (much like the case with former chronic alcoholics or former cocaine or heroin addicts).** Relapses are most apt to occur during negative emotional states within the first few months after quitting.

In general, the following suggestions and approach to smoking cessation have proven helpful:

1. **Consider the importance of quitting and list the health hazards of smoking and the important reasons for quitting.** Enlist the help of others—especially family and friends—to give moral support, and ask them to avoid smoking in your presence. It may be helpful to work with friends or join groups who are trying to quit smoking. **List locations and situations where and when you are most apt to smoke, and be prepared either to avoid these circumstances or to cope with them.** Each day check the reasons for quitting. Then designate a date on which to quit, preferably a day when your stress level is low and you face few problems and pressures.

2. **Stopping abruptly seems to be more effective than cutting down gradually. Throw away all cigarettes and matches. The use of Zyban (bupropion, Wellbutrin), an antidepressant, has proved especially valuable in some smokers because this reduces the desire to smoke, even in persons who are not depressed. Zyban may be effective alone, but more commonly, it is administered in conjunction with a nicotine replacement.** It requires a prescription, and the dose and schedule for use should be left to your physician.

   Nicotine replacement may be especially helpful in heavy smokers who are addicted. Nicotine transdermal patches (such as Habitrol, Nicoderm, and Prostep) offer significant advantages over nicotine chewing gum (Nicorette): the former products are easier to use, cause fewer side effects, and deliver a more constant and adequate dose of nicotine. Although nicotine patches can be obtained without a prescription, you should consult your physician regarding dose schedules, especially when the patches are used in combination with Zyban. Other forms of nicotine delivery—by means of a nasal spray or inhaler, for example—appear to be much less effective than patches and chewing gums containing nicotine. You should not smoke if you are using nicotine replacement because smoking might elevate significantly the nicotine concentration in the blood and cause problems, especially in those with heart disease. Anecdotal reports suggesting that nicotine patches may cause heart irregularities and even heart attacks or strokes have caused concern; however, a study of male volunteers revealed no difference in side effects between subjects using nicotine patches and those using patches without nicotine.

   The value of hypnosis and acupuncture is poorly substantiated as a means of smoking cessation, although some have benefited from these treatments.

3. **Be prepared to cope with the urge to smoke, which is especially strong initially during withdrawal.** Changing routine activities may be very helpful. **Perform activities to divert your attention, such as exercising, taking a walk immediately after meals, going to a movie, joining friends who are strongly opposed to smoking, chewing ordinary gum, eating celery or carrot sticks or unsalted pretzels, or sucking on Tic-Tacs.** Avoid substituting high-calorie foods for cigarettes because smoking cessation decreases the body's metabolism and leads to a tendency to gain weight.

Continually recall the health hazards of smoking, including death from heart and lung disease, stroke, a variety of cancers, and risks to the fetus during pregnancy. Some smokers may be helped by formal cessation programs with group interaction and mutual support. While attempting to stop smoking, counseling by telephone ("Quit Lines") are available in some states and may give helpful support and encouragement to "kick the habit" and remain smoke free. You always must remember that the key depends almost entirely on the strength of your desire to quit! **If you fail to quit on the first attempt, try again. From failure, you may learn how to be successful. Remember: two-thirds of those who repeatedly try to quit eventually succeed!**

RISKS of Using Illicit and Some Prescription Drugs

It is impossible to assess accurately the severity and extent of damage to the lives of so many caused by the use of illicit (unlawful) drugs in our nation. Illicit drugs have damaged or destroyed the lives of countless adults; however, of great concern is the devastating influence the use of these drugs has on our adolescent children. Illicit drugs frequently lead to antisocial and sometimes violent behavior and serious or fatal injuries. The prevalence of illicit drug use in our schools is shocking, but more frightening is the frequent inability to control effectively this very serious scourge in our society.

The following information is derived partly from *The Teen Health Book: A Parent's Guide to Adolescent Health and Well-Being*, by Ralph I. Lopez, M.D. The author is a highly competent pediatrician with special expertise in the treatment of teenagers. His book is a valuable resource for all parents.

Marijuana ("Pot," "Grass," "Weed," "Hash")

Some would have us believe that marijuana is a harmless drug that should be legalized and used recreationally because it provides a pleasurable state of euphoria or "high" ("an exaggerated feeling of physical and mental well-being that is not justified by external reality") that lasts for several hours. **But marijuana smoke contains toxic compounds, including carbon monoxide, and possibly more cancer-causing chemicals than cigarette smoke. Lung irritation and a cough often are experienced. Marijuana is sometimes contaminated with another illicit drug such as phencyclidine (PCP) or treated with "embalming fluid" to enhance its euphoric effect. This adulteration of marijuana can cause severe harmful effects.**

There is some evidence that the active ingredient of marijuana (a chemical, tetrahydrocannabinol [THC]) may depress the immune system and decrease the defense mechanism against infec-

tion. Recent studies reveal that smoking "pot" regularly depletes chemicals (antioxidants) in the lungs that protect against heart disease and lung cancer. Marijuana, which reaches its full effect in 10 to 30 minutes, can increase the heart rate and blood pressure and may affect some of the body's hormones. **THC concentrates in brain fat and other body fat, and it takes up to 4 weeks for a single dose to be eliminated from the body. It impairs learning and short-term memory and affects the ability to stay focused on a subject. Especially serious is marijuana's ability to distort judgment and to delay reaction time and coordination, causing a significant number of automobile crashes with serious injuries and fatalities. It has been estimated that 45% of reckless drivers, not impaired by alcohol, test positive for marijuana. When alcohol and marijuana use are combined, the possibility of a serious car crash further increases, as both intellectual function and coordination are impaired even more.**

Today marijuana is about 10 times more potent than it was 40 years ago. The average age of a first-time marijuana smoker is about 14 years; half of 12th graders have smoked marijuana, and about one of four of these students uses it regularly. **Therefore, it is very important that parents, pediatricians, and counselors intervene and try to prevent use of this drug by appropriate educational efforts in school before children reach their teens.**

Recently, there has been a trend to smoke marijuana that has been soaked in formaldehyde (embalming fluid) and then dried. This can cause a rapid heart rate, tremulousness, sweating, excess salivation, agitation, disorganized speech and thoughts, diminished attention, weakness, convulsions, and coma. These effects are quite similar to those caused by PCP, discussed later. Marijuana soaked with embalming fluid has been given many names in different parts of the nation (e.g., illie, sherm, wet, hydro, loveboat, happy sticks, and clickers).

Because tolerance to marijuana develops (i.e., the pleasant high sensations associated with smoking become less and less with prolonged use of the drug), the user may smoke more often or turn to other illicit drugs that often are addictive and even more dangerous to health. It seems unconscionable to consider legalization of any drug that can harm our children. Some argue that marijuana should be legalized for medical use because it may be helpful in the treatment of nausea caused by chemotherapy in cancer patients and may stimulate the appetite of patients with AIDS. Although this sounds like a reasonable and compassionate argument, the consensus of most medical experts is that there are legal drugs (including marinol, a THC derivative of marijuana) that are as effective or more effective in treatment of these conditions. **The main concern is that legalization of marijuana, even if only for medical use, would make this substance more available to teenagers and adults and that chronic use of this drug not only impairs achievement in any endeavor but also is a "gateway" to harder illicit drugs.**

Unfortunately, children and teenagers' marijuana use in the United States has continued to increase, and sadly, parents, who should be role models for their children, are also smoking this illicit drug more frequently. One very troubling development is that markedly increased amounts of marijuana are being smuggled across the Canadian border into the United States. Cultivation of marijuana is widespread in parts of Canada, especially British Columbia, where the drug is known as "BC bud." This marijuana is considerably more potent than Mexican varieties. Unfortunately, Canadian laws are much more lenient on those who grow or traffic marijuana.

Persons who question the damaging effects of smoking marijuana should consult the books *Keep Off the Grass* and *Marijuana and Medicine*, written and edited by Gabriel G. Nahas, MD, PhD, an international authority on the subject.

Although less frequently used than marijuana, some of the following illicit drugs are particularly dangerous to use because they may cause very serious reactions or death.

Hallucinogens

Another category of illicit drugs are the hallucinogens, which include LSD (lysergic acid diethylamide), PCP ("angel dust"), mescaline, and psilocybin.

- *LSD* ("acid") can cause a frightening "trip" with slurred speech, elevated blood pressure and heart rate, dilated pupils, blurred vision, increased body temperature, sweating, hallucinations (distorted feelings, images, and unreal beliefs), loss of reality, and dangerous behavior that can result in severe injury or death (e.g., trying to "fly" out of a window). There may be permanent brain damage and recurrent visual "flashbacks" of the experience caused by the drug that may last for years and cause extreme fear and anxiety. A "bad trip," which refers to an unpleasant experience caused by the drug, frequently occurs with LSD. Memory may be impaired and attention span reduced.
- *Mescaline* (derived from a cactus), although much weaker than LSD, causes some of the same manifestations as LSD: increased body temperature, heart rate, and blood pressure with dilated pupils and disorientation; however, the trip is said to be easier to manage and there is usually no sense of panic.
- *Phencyclidine* ("angel dust") can cause a loss of inhibitions, with euphoria, can impair judgment and distort thinking, and may cause violent behavior, which may be dangerous to the user and others. However, its effect is unpredictable. In addition to hallucinations, PCP can increase blood pressure and heart rate and can induce sweating and flushing. Muscle rigidity, impaired speech, visual disturbances, convulsions, delirium, and paranoia (feeling of persecution) may occur. Embalming fluid has been

used to cover the smell of PCP to evade detection through customs.

- *Psilocybin* ("mushrooms" or "shrooms"), found in some mushrooms, can cause hallucinations within a few minutes that last for up to 12 hours. The individual may appear drunk and experience nausea, muscle cramps, and abdominal pain. The associated disorientation may result in severe or fatal injuries. When the effects of psilocybin have worn off, the individual may become very depressed and fall into a deep sleep.

Stimulants

Another category of illicit drugs includes amphetamine, methamphetamine, cocaine, and ecstasy.

- *Amphetamine* ("speed") produces a sense of exhilaration and a mind-altering effect that can be very pleasurable. The heart rate and blood pressure are increased and pupils dilated. However, too much amphetamine may cause a psychotic state (mental disorder with a change in personality) with hallucinations, delusions, and paranoid feelings (a belief that people are making derogatory remarks about you or are conspiring against you). Unfortunately, certain prescription drugs (Ritalin and Aderall), which are not amphetamines and are administered for treatment of attention deficit disorder (ADD), have been misused by some students to obtain effects similar to those obtained from amphetamine.
- *Methamphetamine* ("speed," "ice"), similar to amphetamine, is more powerful, and with chronic use, it can severely damage and destroy parts of the brain. The loss of a memory center in the brain may be comparable to the destruction seen in Alzheimer's disease. Amphetamine and methamphetamine cause a sense of well-being and rarely may cause hallucinations, and they can increase heart and breathing rates and blood pressure. Methamphetamine makes the user feel bold and powerful,

and this may result in violent behavior. Methamphetamine-related crimes and arrests have increased markedly. Side effects of diarrhea, loss of bladder control, suppression of appetite, and insomnia may occur. Occasionally, these drugs cause psychotic episodes, a condition in which the individual is mentally deranged and loses contact with reality. Withdrawal from amphetamines may cause what is known as "crashing" with a feeling of severe depression, which requires antidepressants and psychotherapy. Although the use of many other illicit drugs has declined, recently, there has been a marked increase in the use of methamphetamine in rural as well as urban areas. It is reported that 1 in 14 teenagers have used the drug. A clue to the chronic use of methamphetamine is its damaging effect on teeth, which become eroded and destroyed. This is known as "Meth Mouth." Chronic use of methamphetamine (whether smoked, inhaled, eaten, or taken intravenously) causes a very dry mouth and severe tooth destruction, but there is not much pain associated with the tooth decay. The loss of teeth and the need for dentures has been increasing, even in young persons using the drug. As might be expected, Meth Mouth is particularly prevalent in prisoners who have used the drug for prolonged periods before imprisonment.

Increased use of this drug has been attributed to readily available over-the-counter drugs that contain pseudoephedrine, which can be used to make crystal methamphetamine. Some states are limiting the sale of drugs containing pseudoephedrine unless there are adequate indications for its use. It is well said that methamphetamine's "stimulating effect and erasure of inhibitions contribute to sex marathons that have increased the spread of HIV." The appearance of a recent HIV strain, which is resistant to all medications used to control this deadly virus, may partly be due to use of methamphetamine and frequent sexual exposure to multiple partners without the protection of a condom. Sadly, babies born to methamphetamine users are also addicted to this devastating drug.

- *Cocaine* ("coke," "snow," "flake") produces a euphoria that is similar to an amphetamine high with increased energy, movement, and speech. The user senses a feeling of power and confidence. Altering cocaine with baking powder creates "crack" ("rock," "base," "white tornado"), a cheaper form of cocaine that is more addictive, more powerful, and more dangerous. Users may become hyperactive, psychotic, and paranoid (suspiciousness, sense of being persecuted, delusions of grandeur). Interest in food, sex, or surroundings may disappear, and mood swings may occur. Cocaine can cause dilated pupils, confusion with slurred speech, and pronounced increases in heart rate and blood pressure and may be accompanied by strokes, seizures, heart attack, and respiratory failure. After this drug's use, a crash occurs, at which time the user feels terrible, irritable, and fatigued and craves more of the drug. One in four car collisions with fatalities of drivers between ages 16 and 45 years is related to use of cocaine or a combination of cocaine and alcohol.
- *Crank* ("chasing the dragon") is a heroin–crack combination that prolongs the euphoria of crack and lessens the crash that follows its use. Cocaine, crack, and crank addicts frequently resort to violent crime to obtain money to support the cost of these drugs, which they constantly crave. Cocaine withdrawal with rehabilitation is essential. Cocaine Anonymous programs may be helpful.

Case Report

When only 14 years old, N.D. smoked marijuana daily with high school classmates. Much of the time he was "stoned" from the excess use of this illicit drug. He was the son of a single mother who had no influence and little interest in curbing his use of marijuana. His performance in school was dismal, and he showed no interest in any sports activities. By the age of 15 years, he had dropped out of school and had begun smoking increased amounts of marijuana because lesser quantities did not provide the pleasure initially experienced.

By the age of 17 years, he had switched to snorting cocaine, which provided a high that was greater and far more pleasurable than marijuana. However, this caused severe addiction and required chronic use to prevent unpleasant withdrawal symptoms. To furnish his chronic need for cocaine, he became involved as a supplier of cocaine to support his own use. This led to his arrest when he was 19 years old and to imprisonment for 5 years.

When N.D. was released at the age of 24 years, he immediately returned to using cocaine, and one evening, consumption of excess alcohol combined with cocaine resulted in coma and death. During hospitalization, he was discovered to have a hepatitis virus that may have resulted from sharing a contaminated needle that was used for injecting cocaine into a vein. Sadly, this sequence of marijuana serving as a "gateway" drug to more serious and addictive illicit drugs is extremely common. Legalization of marijuana could have a devastating effect on a large segment of our children.

- *Ecstasy* ("E," "x," "XTC," "ADAM") is a methamphetamine-like substance that currently is very popular among teenagers and college students. It causes euphoria (a great sense of well-being) but may interfere with brain function and impair memory and coordination. Users may experience anxiety and decreased appetite, although they usually remain fairly alert and aware of their surroundings. The drug elevates blood pressure and heart rate and dilates pupils. A day or two after ingesting ecstasy, a period of exhaustion occurs. Although it is not addictive, ecstasy is a very dangerous drug that kills some of its users. Whether a permanent disturbance of brain function occurs is not yet known.
- *Khat* (pronounced cot) chewing khat leaves or buds for its stimulating and euphoric effects is particularly popular in Africa, where its use is permitted freely; however, in the United States, it is illegal. The stimulating effect is quite similar to amphetamine (which it resembles chemically) or to small amounts of

cocaine. It is an addictive substance that is popular among immigrants, especially from Yemen, Somalia, and Ethiopia, and it is becoming increasingly available in the United States. Khat may suppress appetite, elevate blood pressure and heart rate, and cause intense thirst, insomnia, irritability, hallucinations, psychosis, sweating, stomach ulcers, impotence, constipation, urinary retention, and inflammation and cancer of the mouth and esophagus. It also may disrupt a normal pregnancy and interfere with some medications. As with other illicit drugs, khat should be avoided, not only because it is illegal, but also because of the serious health consequences of this substance.

- *Betel nuts* Finally, chewing betel nuts presents still another unhealthy and potentially serious practice. Chewing betel nuts as an herbal medicine and for their stimulating and euphoric effects is especially popular in India and Asia, where they are used like chewing tobacco. Their use is legal, and they are now being chewed by a significant number of immigrants and their associates in other countries. This practice can damage the teeth and mouth, causing cancer of the mouth, throat, and esophagus. It also can increase heart rate, blood pressure, respiration, sweating, and temperature and may cause seizures (convulsions), blurred vision, and paralysis. In addition, these nuts may bring about allergic reactions and undesirable interactions with medications. Because of the side effects and possible serious complications, there is no reason or excuse for chewing betel nuts.

Inhalants

Model glue, nail-polish remover, some cleaning fluids, aerosols and hair sprays, gasoline, kerosene, freon (used in air conditioners), butane gas, lighter fluid, paint thinners, and typewriter correction fluids are sometimes inhaled by young persons (7 to 17 years old) to obtain a high—an intoxicating and stimulating effect. Because they cannot buy alcohol or cigarettes, children and teenagers sometimes experiment with inhalants. This practice may cause drunkenness with slurred speech and a loss of consciousness and even suffocation. This dangerous practice can result in severe anemia, brain and liver damage, and sudden "sniffing" death. Professional help is important to prevent continuation of this practice.

- *Amyl nitrite* ("poppers," "liquid gold"), which was administered in the past by physicians to relieve heart pain (angina), occasionally is used by teenagers to obtain the exhilarating, euphoric sensation that this drug causes when inhaled. This and similar drugs dilate blood vessels and can cause a drop in the blood pressure and, if swallowed, can be fatal.
- *Whippet*, an amyl nitrate, may be obtained in supermarkets in canisters containing a propellant to make seltzer water. The propellant can be collected by inflating a balloon and then inhaled to produce a brief high. This may result in respiratory depression and sudden death.

Sedatives

- *Ketamine* ("vitamin K," "ketaject," "special K"), a relative of PCP, causes an anaesthetic effect and can cause hallucinations. It may result in loss of consciousness and is considered a "date rape drug".
- *GHB* (gamma-hydroxybutyrate, also known as "liquid ecstasy" or "G") is another dangerous "date rape drug" that is odorless, tasteless, and colorless. Only a few drops can cause relaxation, sedation, and deep sleep. Respiratory depression, followed by coma, and sometimes death can occur. Unfortunately, butyrolactone and butanediol, which produce GHB when ingested, are available for purchase on the internet.
- *Rohypnol* ("Roofies"), a powerful sedative from the same family of drugs as Valium, has been used for insomnia. Because the user usually cannot recall what occurred after taking this sedative, it also has been called a "date rape drug".

One of eight female college students reported that she was the victim of a date rape; however, alcohol was present in the blood of 80% of date-rape victims. Marijuana was present in 30%, whereas ketamine and rohypnol each were found in only 3%.

To avoid or minimize the possibility of rape, it is strongly recommended that a woman always be accompanied by a friend or escort when entering a bar, tavern, or night club, and a woman should never drink alone with a stranger. It is especially important that drinks never be left out of view, for example, to go dancing or to go to the ladies' room. A drug can easily be added to a drink that is left unattended without affecting the taste. Be aware that a drink with a drug can easily replace a normal (undrugged) drink if they are not kept in constant view.

- *Klonopin* is a prescription drug that is similar in action to "roofies" and is administered for the treatment of anxiety. Also, it has been taken as a drug of abuse to enhance the effect of opiates.
- *Barbiturates* are depressants ("downers") that physicians sometimes administer for sedation, to calm anxious or psychotic persons. Like alcohol, they impair coordination and judgment. The excess user appears drunk. Their addictive properties require careful withdrawal, sometimes necessitating hospitalization or a detoxification center.
- *Quaaludes* ("ludes") also are powerful sedatives that are occasionally taken, mainly by college students, in place of barbiturates. These drugs are dangerous, and an overdose can be fatal, especially when combined with alcoholic beverages.

Opiates

Opiates (also called narcotics) or opiate-like substances are sometimes abused as illicit drugs.

- *Opium* is rarely used in the United States.
- *Morphine* is derived from opium and is administered as a pain killer.

- *Heroin* ("smack," "junk," "black tar," "China white," "horse") is a modified form of morphine that affects the brain faster than other opiates.
- *Codeine* is a pain killer and is often combined with Tylenol.
- *Dextromethorphan*, a codeine derivative, is a cough suppressant.
- *Methadone* can be used as a substitute for heroin, and it can be taken by mouth.

In the past few years, the use of heroin has increased markedly in the United States and often has led to violent crime to support the cost of the drug for those addicted. Heroin addicts are unable to function effectively and to hold a job. Use of methadone, instead of heroin, usually enables those individuals to function in society and to return to a gainful occupation; however, regrettably, they then remain addicted to methadone.

All of these drugs are highly addictive when given in large doses. They can be injected into a vein or taken orally. They may cause sedation, slow and irregular heartbeat, respiratory failure, stroke, heart attack, nausea, vomiting, constricted pupils, and coma. Severe withdrawal symptoms (shaking, sweating, stomach cramps, muscle aches, chills, diarrhea, vomiting, running nose, and eyes) occur when the drugs are withheld. Addicts frequently die of an overdose. Infection with HIV, hepatitis virus, and other germs is common in those injecting drugs into their veins.

Placement in a detoxification center, followed by in-patient care, is usually essential for treatment of addiction. Ultimately, care in a "halfway" program is required to follow the patient closely before returning home and further treatment. Support of friends who do not use drugs or from those who have undergone successful drug rehabilitation or support groups such as NA (Narcotics Anonymous) may be very helpful.

Steroids, Creatine, DHEAs (dehydroepiandrosterone sulfate)

- *Steroids:* Less than 12 years ago, the National Institute on Drug Abuse estimated that 262,000 students in grades 7 through 12 used anabolic steroids illegally to build muscle strength for competitive athletics. **Recently, a survey reported that up to 1 million teenagers use steroids (or androstenedione, which is converted in the body to steroids) each year; the majority are boys who take steroids, not to improve their athletic ability, but to build a muscular body and enhance their appearance.** This is very regrettable; athletic performance, winning, and muscular appearance are not worth the risk of damaging one's health. **Steroids can be harmful and cause stunted growth, fluid retention, elevated blood pressure, elevated blood sugar, liver disease, decreased good cholesterol (HDL), heart damage, increased irritability, aggressiveness, violent behavior ('roid rage), depression, psychosis, and suicide. In males, the breasts become enlarged. Testicular size and function decrease, and male hormone production and sperm formation are reduced. In females, the voice may deepen. Breasts diminish in size. The development of eggs and ovulation is inhibited, and menstruation is disrupted.**

- *Androstenedione* is a natural male hormone, secreted by the adrenal glands that can be obtained over-the-counter (without a prescription). This hormone, banned in the Olympics, became especially popular with teenagers when several famous professional baseball players revealed that they were taking it. However, it can impair growth and sexual development and can cause testicular shrinkage in males and growth of undesirable body hair in females.

  Substances used to increase sports performance and body building are reported to be the "largest-growing segment of the $18 billion dietary supplement industry." It has been reported that 50% of professional baseball players are taking steroids, and about 80% use stimulants periodically.

- *Creatine* is a combination of amino acids (chemicals that build proteins) that are thought to build muscle mass with physical training. It is not an illicit (unlawful) substance, and creatine has become exceedingly popular; many professional and amateur athletes use it, although there is no conclusive evidence that it enhances muscle mass and physical strength. **Whether creatine may affect health is not yet known, but because it increases the workload of the kidneys, it never should be taken by individuals with impaired kidney function or by diabetics or older persons.** It may cause some abdominal discomfort.
- *DHEA* is a steroid that builds body mass, but it should be avoided; side effects are similar to androstenedione.

Finally, it is important to avoid using herbs about which little is known. Some of these may be dangerous to your health and safety. *Salvia divinorum* can be smoked and chewed. It is used in Mexico and is being smoked and chewed by some American teenagers and young adults "in search of mind-bending experiences." It can cause hallucinations that alter reality and distort what you feel and see. The Drug Enforcement Administration may eventually declare this an illegal substance. Some of the effects or complications of illicit drugs are indicated in **Figure 10**.

Illicit drug use in the United States represents an enormous problem for everyone, especially teenagers. In 1960, fewer than 1% of American teenagers had tried marijuana or other illicit drugs; however, by 1980, more than 60% had taken illicit drugs, and 10% of high school seniors were "stoned" every day. About 40% of teenagers used alcohol or drugs at parties. Illicit drug use, particularly marijuana and ecstasy, continues to increase in our nation.

It is very important for parents to recognize manifestations of illicit drug and alcohol use by their children. The following signs are often present: antisocial, withdrawn, secretive, aggressive, and sometimes violent behavior; failing school grades; a decreased con-

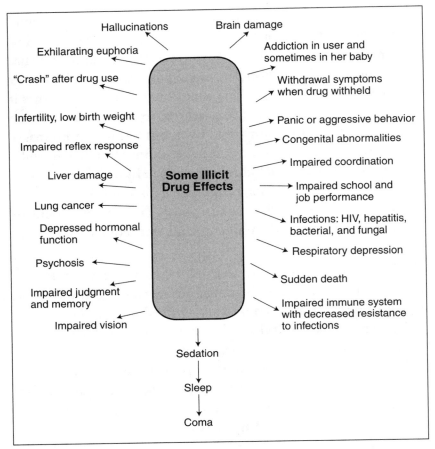

Figure 10. Some effects and complications that may be caused by illicit drugs.

centration and attention span; a lack of interest in surroundings, sports, and food; lying and stealing; mood swings with highs followed by depression; sedation; drunkenness; stoned and slurred speech; dilated pupils; and frequent injuries.

Interdiction and appropriate criminal prosecution are, of course, necessary to combat the use of illegal drugs. In addition, treatment, rehabilitation, and support programs are essential

for those dependent on illicit drugs or alcohol; however, the key to combating most effectively the use of illicit drugs and alcohol is *prevention*. The National Center on Addiction and Drug Substance Abuse at Columbia University has reported the following: "Based on everything we know, a young man or woman who gets to age twenty-one without smoking, abusing alcohol, or using illegal drugs is virtually certain never to do so."

There can be no improvement on *The Twelve Key Guiding Principles For Parents*, which "NYC—Parents in Action" set forth in their publication: *Focus—A Practical Parenting Guide*:

1. "**Start early** to instill values and give accurate information to children about the dangers of drug use. Prepare them well in advance for the time when they may be asked to try tobacco, alcohol, and drugs.

2. **Speak up. Take a stand.** Don't be an enabler. If anyone or anything encourages your children to try alcohol, tobacco, or drugs, take action!

3. **Remember that you are a role model for your child.** Actions speak louder than words. If you abuse alcohol or drugs, your child is very likely to become an abuser.

4. **Take advantage of every teachable moment.** Use news stories, television, and movies as opportunities to discuss drugs and alcohol.

5. **Reinforce both the information and the rules you teach your children.** Repetition is key to learning.

6. **Know what is going on in your child's life at home, in school, and with friends.** Listen to your child and to your child's friends.

7. **Know the attitudes towards drug and alcohol use your child may be learning** from babysitters, day care providers, camp counselors, family friends, and relatives.

8. **Set limits and adhere to them.** Be firm and consistent for your child's sake. Stand by your family's rules.

9. **Learn the tell-tale signs of drug and alcohol abuse.**

10 **Take action if you believe or have evidence that your child is trying drugs or alcohol.** Do something about it. Don't wait for the problem to go away by itself.

11. **Keep in touch with the parents of your child's friends.** Work together with other parents to establish curfews and other rules for all your children.

12. **Remember, parent power is stronger than peer pressure.** No one loves your child as much as you do. Your love for your child and your determination to help your child stay drug and alcohol free are powerful weapons in the fight against drug abuse." (Reproduced with permission from NYC—Parents In Action.)

Almost all parents agree that nothing is more important than the health and welfare of their children. Appropriate guidance regarding healthy lifestyle, starting at preschool and kindergarten ages, can be enormously helpful for future generations. At times, parents may become extremely concerned and enraged by the irresponsible action of their children; however, it usually is most effective to remain calm and provide constructive criticism, supported by accurate knowledge, in a firm but controlled and mature manner. It is extremely important to have basic information about illicit drugs when offering parental advice and guidance; opinions without knowledge can be disastrous. Patience is virtue, and it is usually best to avoid being overly critical and judgmental when dealing with drug problems in teenagers.

RISKS of Sexually Transmitted Disease

Smart sex avoids any chance of sexually transmited disease (STD). STDs, including AIDS, are increasing yearly in the United States and elsewhere. There are now 2 million Americans with HIV infection. **Most STDs (gonorrhea, chlamydia, syphilis, and genital warts) and their complications, such as PID (pelvic inflammatory disease), usually can be treated successfully. However, there are no cures for AIDS, genital herpes, or hepatitis B. The risk of cervical cancer is higher in women who have had multiple sexual partners or in women whose partners have had multiple sexual partners.** The risk also is increased in women who have HIV, human papilloma virus (HPV), or genital warts.

It is not the intent of this book to discuss the diagnosis and treatment of STDs. Management should be left to the physicians who see individuals with any manifestations of these diseases, such as the following: pus-like discharge from the penis or vagina; burning or frequency of urination; painful or painless sores on the genitalia, rectum, tongue, or lips; lower abdominal pain in women; testicular pain; venereal warts; joint pains with fever; swollen lymph nodes in the groins; unexplained sore throat; or conjunctivitis. **Chlamydia, rarely recognized 20 years ago, is now the most commonly reported infection in the United States; because it can infect the eye, it is the most common cause of blindness worldwide.**

Women with chlamydial or gonorrheal infections sometimes show no evidence of disease. Therefore, if their male sexual partner has been diagnosed with either of these diseases, it is always important to check repeatedly for any evidence of gonorrhea or chlamydia in the female.

Of vital importance for all Americans is to understand what behavior puts them and their family at risk for developing infection with HIV. AIDS is invariably a deadly disease. Although there are drugs that are helpful in suppressing the disease, no cure and no vaccine can prevent the disease.

Parents must learn as much as possible about STDs; they should understand how HIV is transmitted and how to avoid these infections. They should convey this information to teenagers, who are often confused about STDs, and to young children at an appropriate age. **Sex education may start in schools as early as the third grade. Emphasis should be on prevention.**

It is reported that 25% of STDs in the United States occur in teenagers and that 45% of White girls 15 to 19 years old have had intercourse; the percentage increases to 56% in other races. The percentages of males having intercourse is even higher. It is reported that 16% of high school sophomores have had four or more sexual partners, and one in four sexually active teenagers will contract a STD. **Another very disturbing statistic is that 20% of sexually active girls between 15 and 19 years old become pregnant each year; the United States has the highest rate of teenage pregnancy in the industrialized world.**

About 25% of all new HIV cases occur under the age of 21 years, and nearly 1 in 10 children will lose their virginity before the age of 13 years. Some 15% of teenagers have genital warts, and girls ages 15 to 19 years old with genital warts have high rates of gonorrhea. About 50% of teenagers between 13 and 19 have had oral sex. These shocking statistics emphasize the risks of STD in our children and the importance of competent educational efforts regarding risky and safe sex. A study reported in the journal *Pediatrics* indicates that girls with high self-esteem are more likely to abstain, whereas boys with high self-esteem are more likely to engage in sex.

Some research on teenage sex suggests that, if a program of sex education favors abstinence but still stresses the importance of pro-

129

tection from STDs, sexual activity does not increase; teenagers often postpone sex. One study revealed that teenage daughters of mothers who disapproved of their having sex were more likely to remain virgins longer than teenage daughters of mothers who did not disapprove of them having sex.

Abstinence is the surest protection from STDs. However, the employment of a latex condom is invaluable in the prevention of STDs, including HIV. Unfortunately, men and teenage boys often will not use a condom. A recent survey indicated that 400,000 students reported incidents of unprotected sex while drinking alcohol. Today, females purchase one third of the condoms. Having a female partner apply a condom to an erect penis can be more acceptable to the male.

It must be appreciated that oral sex carries the same risk as vaginal intercourse. The following have been reported to increase the risk of infection with HIV:

1. Intercourse without a condom
2. Intercourse with multiple partners
3. Injection of illicit drugs with a shared needle (It has been reported one third of AIDS cases are drug related.)
4. Sexual contact with persons who inject illicit drugs
5. Intercourse with drug and alcohol abusers who often are irresponsible and do not use a condom
6. Intercourse with a partner who has other STDs
7. A needle prick after drawing blood from a person with HIV
8. Blood transfusion (rare today because of careful screening for HIV)
9. Sodomy (anal intercourse) is particularly risky because bleeding may occur and infect a partner

Because infection with HIV can lead to the development of AIDS, which is invariably fatal, any of the sex practices listed previously must be avoided. Nothing is more dangerous than promiscuity (having sexual intercourse with multiple partners) without a condom—it is like playing Russian roulette. A condom should *always* be used during sexual intercourse unless it is absolutely certain through adequate testing that the partners ("straight" or "gay") are uninfected. **Risky sex should never be an option, as it may cost you your life!** Regrettably, an alarming number (about 50%) of male college students use condoms incorrectly and thus increase the risk of STDs and unintended pregnancies.

Abstinence is always the best choice, as it guarantees safety from STDs, pregnancy, and their emotional consequences. It is likely that abstinence and educational programs will be more accepted by some than others. Therefore, providing detailed educational information about the use of a condom and its protective value is only reasonable. Counseling teenagers and adults regarding the dangers of STDs has not been particularly effective; nevertheless, the crucial importance **of using a condom for protection must be emphasized and re-emphasized.** It is extremely important for health workers to contact males and females who are known to have HIV or AIDS in an effort to minimize the spread of infection. However, contacting infected individuals who are known to have HIV or AIDS is becoming increasingly more difficult. Reportedly, men now find "casual sex partners on the Internet, bypassing bars and central meeting places where public health workers traditionally have reached people" infected with this deadly virus.

Safety Measures to Prevent Injury and Some Diseases

The keys to safety and injury prevention are knowledge, anticipation, and preventive action. It has been reported that unintentional injury is the leading cause of death of individuals 1 to 34 years old; however, most injuries can be prevented. One might assume that common sense will protect us from most injuries, yet as Voltaire observed, "Common sense is not so common."

Most adults are aware of numerous ways to avoid injuries. It is crucial, however, that parents be constantly vigilant regarding injuries that could happen to their children. *Anticipating the possibility of an injury before it happens is the key.* Some evidence suggests that stress, depression, and anxiety may be responsible for certain individuals being injury prone. Apparently, emotional problems can interfere with an individual's ability to focus and concentrate on avoiding injuries.

Safety on the Road

Automobiles

Car crashes and serious injuries are so common that they should be discussed, at least briefly, in connection with lifestyles, as intelligence, anticipation, and proper precautions can save lives. Precautions to prevent serious injuries and fatalities are self-evident to most individuals. However, young adults and teenagers, in particular, frequently seem unconcerned with danger and the possible consequences of careless behavior, and they often do not take any precautions to use safety equipment to prevent injury. Drugs and alcohol serve only to augment this false sense of immortality and careless behavior.

We all should realize that reckless, aggressive driving and speeding in a vehicle, especially when the driver is under the influence of alcohol and/or illicit drugs, are responsible for the greatest

number of car-crash deaths in our nation each year. *Never* drive under the influence of alcohol or illicit drugs, and *never* ride with a driver who has been drinking or using illicit drugs! Furthermore, as we all know, it is very dangerous to drive while very tired or while taking prescription drugs that cause fatigue. Individuals with a history of seizures or "blackouts" should consult a physician regarding the risk of driving a vehicle. **Safe driving can best be achieved by driving "defensively"—that is, carefully, under control, without excessive speed, and remaining mentally alert and prepared to respond promptly to avoid collisions that are often fatal. One should *always* remain focused on driving and not be distracted by the activities of others in the car or by the use of a cellular phone or simply day dreaming and not concentrating.** Wet or icy roads and those covered by snow, wet leaves, or oil are always particularly hazardous and require slow driving without sudden braking to minimize the chance of skidding and crashing. Tire pressure should be checked approximately every 3,000 miles, which is about the time when an oil change is indicated. Although low pressure in tires may give better traction on snow, low pressure makes tires more likely to blow out when driving very rapidly.

It is extremely important to drive slowly and with great caution during the day, and especially at night, in areas where animals may suddenly run across the road. Fatal injuries from car crashes periodically result from attempts to avoid hitting an animal. Also, whenever entering an area of fog, drive very slowly and with great caution. Frequently, fog occurs in patches, and it is dangerous to accelerate between patches. Turn on the windshield wipers and defroster to remove moisture from the windshield and to improve visibility. If your car has fog lights, turn them on and use low-beam headlights, as high beams can reflect fog and impair visibility.

One very tragic example of the great danger of driving through fog occurred on route I-75 in Tennessee in 1990. Serious collisions had occurred previously on this stretch of highway because of fog, and illuminated signs had been installed to warn drivers of the hazards of fog in this area. Unfortunately, the sign to alert drivers traveling north was malfunctioning and not illuminated or flashing, and most vehicles continued to proceed at 50 to 70 miles per hour. With the sudden appearance of very dense fog, visibility was almost totally lost. At that point, lack of visibility made it impossible to avoid collisions by vehicles entering the fog, and this led immediately to a chain of crashes involving about 100 vehicles; 12 persons lost their lives. Perhaps the lesson for all of us who drive is to remember that fog on a highway can be extremely hazardous, as it can markedly and suddenly impair visibility. The importance of driving very slowly and with great caution through foggy areas cannot be overemphasized, because these precautions may save your life.

Strong winds present a special hazard, because the force of a strong wind may cause a driver to lose control of a vehicle (especially "high-riding" SUVs, vans, and trucks) and result in a collision. The best way to avoid a crash when the wind is strong is to drive very slowly. The National Highway Traffic Safety Administration recently demonstrated that more than one third of SUVs have a tendency to roll over. They estimated that of the 4,451 persons who died in SUV crashes, roll-overs occurred in about 61% of the fatal crashes.

Icy, wet, and snow-covered roads are treacherous and responsible for an enormous number of serious injuries and fatalities. With icy road conditions, driving any vehicle is extremely hazardous and should be avoided unless absolutely essential. A driver should also remember that snow or water on the road of a bridge is often the first to freeze and may be especially slippery. **Driving very slowly and with great caution is, of course, the best way to minimize a car crash and injury. If you have to stop suddenly in a car that has antilock brakes, it is best to step on the brake and maintain**

pressure; pumping the brake defeats the effectiveness of anti-lock brakes. Pumping the brakes of cars made before 1990 is justified, as they do not have antilock brakes. Today, most cars have antilock brakes. In heavy snow conditions, it is best to operate a vehicle with all-wheel drive as this provides greater tire traction and helps prevent skidding.

Frank Niland, a professional driving instructor, makes several important suggestions that can improve driving safety. He recommends that:

1. Gripping the steering wheel at 8 and 4 o'clock provides better control than gripping the wheel at 9 and 3 o'clock. The latter encourages "hand-over-hand steering" and greater instability, especially on slippery roads. Holding the wheel at 8 and 4 o'-clock allows the driver to "push and pull" the wheel for turning without "hand-over-hand steering." Furthermore, if your arms are crossed during a collision, inflation of an air bag may force your forearms into your face.

2. Place the gear in neutral to slow the car during a skid without braking. This may improve braking on ice, as in the neutral position, the wheels driving your car stop rotating, which provides greater stability. During a skid, placing the transmission in neutral may enable you to regain control without using the brakes. Niland recommends doing things slowly and looking and steering in the direction you want to go.

3. Detect black ice (ice that looks like a wet road) by no spray from the road on your windshield. The treacherous nature of black ice is that you cannot distinguish it from wet pavement, especially at night. However, if there is no spray from the road caused by vehicles ahead of you and you don't have to use your windshield wipers, you should assume that the road is icy.

4. In rain, slush, and snow conditions, drive in the tracks of those

vehicles ahead of you for better traction, as these tracks are usually drier and less slippery than elsewhere.

5. Skidding can easily occur on wet asphalt at high speeds and on flooded roads even at slow speeds. A car can hydroplane; that is, car tires can lose contact with the road, resulting in loss of tire traction and skidding.

Finally, it should be emphasized that it is extremely hazardous to repair a flat tire or to seek or offer assistance to a motorist on a highway. Each year people are killed or seriously injured by passing cars while trying to repair their car or assist others. Always have a cell phone in your car, and immediately call 911 and seek professional automobile assistance if your car breaks down or runs out of gas on a highway or heavily trafficked road. It is safest to remain in your vehicle; raising the hood will attract attention and indicates that your car has broken down and that you are in trouble. It can be very helpful if you keep a flashlight in your car to signal at night that you are in distress and need help. Also, keep your headlights on, and turn on your rear flashing lights and interior car lights if you can keep the engine running. Open a window enough to obtain some fresh air, and **if you become stuck in a heavy snow storm, be sure that you prevent the exhaust pipes from becoming blocked by snow, as this could cause a dangerous buildup of carbon monoxide in the car, which could be fatal.** If it is very cold, move your arms and legs frequently to stay warm, and use the car heater as necessary.

Every car owner in the United States, especially those who periodically drive considerable distances from home, should become a member of the American Automobile Association (AAA) to ensure prompt repairs and/or safe transportation, if the car breaks down or a flat tire has to be replaced. Some older persons and those who are frail or ill will need assistance for changing a tire or obtaining help if a car malfunctions.

Case Report

P.R. and three other college students had completed a number of grueling examinations just before spring break. They decided to drive to Florida, where they would spend their vacation together. They had celebrated the night before their departure and stayed up until about 3 A.M.—drinking beer and smoking pot. They got an early start at 8 A.M., as they wanted to drive to Palm Beach (about 1,500 miles away) without stopping. If they took turns driving, this would be possible.

Somewhere in Georgia, the driver apparently fell asleep and the car, traveling at a high speed, veered off the road, struck a tree, and rolled down an embankment. The passenger in the front seat was killed immediately from a broken neck and head injuries, and the students in the back seat were severely injured with multiple fractures, but they survived. The driver was less fortunate, as the severity of his injuries resulted in kidney failure, causing his death several days later.

We do not know whether these students continued to drink beer and smoke pot while driving to Florida, but we do know that none were using seat belts. We assume that they were all too tired to remain alert and wide awake under these circumstances.

These were intelligent, rather typical college students in search of a fun vacation. Yet their extreme fatigue, failure to use seat belts, and probable impairment of judgment, reflexes, and coordination of the driver, perhaps partly from the effects of alcohol and illicit drugs, resulted in a tragic ending that should never have happened.

One should never drive when tired or after consuming alcohol and/or using illicit drugs. The driver must always remain sober and alert. This policy has proved extremely effective in decreasing vehicular crashes in Sweden, where arrest for driving while intoxicated results in mandatory imprisonment for 1 year. We all know the best way to prevent falling asleep while driving is to pull over into a rest area and sleep until adequately rested.

The extreme importance of always being aware of the location of children before moving a car in a driveway or elsewhere cannot be overemphasized. Tragically, a significant number of children are killed by car injuries because they were not visible to the driver. **Young children should, of course, never be left unattended in a vehicle,** and they should be repeatedly warned about hand injuries that can occur from closing car doors; always observe that children are securely seated before closing a door. Whenever driving with young children, it is very important that the driver lock car windows that are accessible to the children. Leaving a young child unattended in a car, even for a few minutes, can result in tragedy. There are reports of severe injuries and fatalities because a child activated a window and was caught and compressed by the window closing. Vigilant parents can prevent such injuries. An infant or young child should never be left alone in a car, as it is always possible that they may injure themselves. Furthermore, prolonged exposure to heat or cold may be severely damaging or even fatal, especially to infants and young children; elevated temperature in a car in very hot weather may cause severe dehydration and death.

The importance of protective helmets, seat belts, and child safety seats is understood by the great majority of adults; nevertheless, too often, employment of these safety devices is overlooked or ignored, which may result in unnecessary injuries and fatalities. Remember that seat belts should be worn at all times, even when traveling short distances, as many car crashes occur only a few miles from home. However, it is recommended that children 8 years of age or younger be placed in child-safety seats; this is the law in some states. Young children and those in child-safety seats must always be secured with seat belts in rear seats of a vehicle.

They never should be permitted to sit in a front seat, as inflation of an air bag can cause severe injury or death of a young child.

Precautions for Other Types of Transportation and Recreation

Protective helmets should be worn by persons using bicycles, motorcycles, mopeds, motorized or nonmotorized scooters, roller blades, downhill skies, snowboards, snowmobiles, sleds, toboggans, ice boats, or any equipment used for sliding down hills on snow, and snow bikes and by anyone learning to ice skate or riding on all-terrain vehicles (ATVs). A rear view mirror attached to the safety helmet is helpful to individuals bicycling or roller blading during the day; however, it is also extremely important for those who bicycle or roller blade on streets at night to wear safety helmets that are equipped with a light on the rear of their helmets, backs, or bicycles. Using reflective tape on the back of clothes and on the rear of a bicycle is also a wise precaution. These simple precautions can reduce the chance of being struck by pursuing vehicles. It also would be wise for individuals to wear safety helmets when riding horses or using skateboards. **It is essential to stress that seat belts and child safety seats be used by adults and children at all times for optimal safety when riding in a vehicle.**

Many injuries can be extremely serious or deadly if one is riding a motorcycle or a moped, as there is no protection from injury except that provided by a helmet. A collision with a motor vehicle is often fatal or leaves the injured permanently incapacitated. **Whenever possible, avoid using a motorcycle for transportation; don't do it! The risk of injury is too great!**

Mopeds, or similar motorized bicycles, are used in many parts of the world because they are relatively inexpensive and/or the use of cars may be limited. They are less dangerous because they do not travel at the high speed of motorcycles. **However, all persons should be given instructions and practice before operating a moped on their own to minimize the possibility of injury.** Many tragic accidents and fatalities have occurred to those who are inexperienced in proper operation and safety measures.

Pedestrians

The great danger of children being struck by a vehicle is a concern of all parents. Nothing is more important than constantly and closely watching young children and carefully guiding them across streets. Children must continually be reminded of the danger of being hit by a car. Teenagers should be repeatedly warned about the dangers of being struck by vehicles while skateboarding and roller skating on streets or "hitching" rides on the rear of buses or trucks. Every effort should be made to prevent these dangerous practices.

Safety on or in the Water

Boating

When boating, it is extremely important to have an adequate number of life jackets immediately available to adults and teenagers. Children and persons who do not know how to swim should wear a life jacket at all times, and children should be closely watched to prevent any possibility of falling overboard. It is strongly recommended that life jackets be used when water skiing or using jet skis.

One of the saddest experiences I am aware of occurred many years ago to a friend of mine. He had spent most of the day with his four young sons cruising off the California coast in his powerboat.

Tragically, no one realized that one of the children had fallen overboard while returning to port. Apparently, the roar of the boat's engine had masked any sound of falling into the ocean and any cries for help. The child was never found. This heart-wrenching experience emphasizes the extreme importance of life jackets and keeping close account of all of those on board the boat. Very young children should always be placed in secure and visible locations. Many states offer boating safety courses.

It should be appreciated that swimming or water skiing, especially in areas where there are many powerboats or jet skis, can be very dangerous. A significant number of serious injuries and deaths occur each year from powerboats striking swimmers that were not seen. **Therefore avoid swimming or water skiing where there is considerable boating activity. It is extremely important to always make sure that the propeller of a powerboat is not rotating when swimmers are nearby or are approaching to board the boat.** This will avoid the possibility of a severe cut from a rotating propeller.

No one who has been drinking alcohol should operate a powerboat. Alcohol can significantly impair judgment, reflexes, and reaction time, which may result in boat collisions with severe injuries and fatalities. **Operating boats at night, or when visibility is reduced by fog, presents a serious risk and requires extreme caution and navigating at a very low speed.** Adequate lights on a boat when navigating in the dark and a fog horn in the presence of thick fog are essential.

The sea can be very treacherous, particularly in stormy weather. Powerful currents running against strong winds can cause huge (rogue) waves that may sometimes reach a height of about 100 feet and can sink small ships. Weather conditions should always be checked before venturing into the ocean. Any evidence of a developing storm should be reason enough to remain on shore. There is always a serious risk that strong winds and currents may carry a small sailboat many miles from shore. It is particularly dangerous to sail a small boat in the ocean far from shore. In time of distress, if you have no shore-to-shore radio to inform the Coast Guard, at least have a cell phone to report immediately if your boat is drifting out to sea. A cell phone should operate if you are within several miles from shore; however, a satellite cell phone may be necessary if you are far from land. A flair gun may also alert others that you need help, particularly at night when you cannot be seen.

Swimming, Diving, and Surfing

When swimming and diving, **it is absolutely essential to know the depth of water before diving or jumping into any body of water.** Severe injuries, particularly to the head, neck, and spinal cord, can occur by diving or jumping into shallow water. Severe neck injuries also may result from diving into ocean surf, especially if the surf is shallow and receding. In the rare event that a swimmer is caught in a strong whirlpool in the ocean, river, or lake, it is best not to become exhausted by repeated unsuccessful attempts to swim away from the suction caused by the whirlpool. It is recommended that, after taking several deep breaths, the swimmer submerge in the whirlpool and then swim away under water, as the suction effect of the whirlpool is lost below the surface of the water.

The undertow, riptides, and currents in the ocean may be a challenge to even the best swimmers so that swimming in the presence of a lifeguard is strongly recommended. **It is extremely important for children, young teenagers, and weak swimmers to remain close to the beach and to avoid swimming in a heavy ocean surf**; this will minimize the chance of getting caught by a strong current and will permit rescue of a swimmer in distress. Currents that pull a swimmer out to sea may be especially difficult to swim against when strong winds increase these currents. In designated swimming areas, danger flags are displayed to warn swimmers when conditions are hazardous. If caught in a powerful current that prevents a swimmer from returning to shore, immediately signal for help; if help is delayed or not available, it is best to swim parallel to the shore, as the current will usually disappear after swimming a few hundred feet. Most important, the swimmers should remain calm and avoid becoming exhausted by swimming against a strong current. No one should risk ocean swimming in a very heavy surf.

Recently, on Long Island, New York, a middle-aged man, who was a good swimmer, was unable to cope with the power of waves and undertow resulting from a subsiding hurricane in the Atlantic Ocean, and he was tossed by the sea against a wall of rocks and sustained fatal head injuries.

Surfing has become an increasingly popular sport on the West and East Coasts of the United States and in Hawaii. Some areas have become very crowded with surfers, and therefore, there is a greater risk of being struck and injured by surfboards in these congested areas. The surfer who is riding a wave is responsible for not striking surfers in the water as he is carried toward the shore. **A leash that attaches the surfboard to the surfer will minimize or prevent a surfboard from striking and injuring others.** Although very few deaths from surfing injuries have been reported, rarely a surfer may be struck in the head and become unconscious and drown. **Another good reason for having a leash attached to your wrist or ankle is that, when a surfer falls into the water, the surfboard will pull the submerged surfer toward the ocean surface.**

Shark Attacks

Although shark attacks are uncommon (70 to 100 attacks annually, resulting in up to 15 deaths worldwide), it is helpful to be familiar with safety suggestions that can minimize attacks in the ocean or connecting waters. George H. Burgess (curator of International Shark Attack File, University of Florida) gives the following advice when swimming or surfing in the ocean:

- Stay in groups, as sharks are more likely to attack an individual swimming alone.
- Stay close to the shore so that you can exit the water quickly and calmly if there is any concern of a shark attack; also, assistance may be more readily available.
- Avoid being in the water during darkness, twilight hours, or early morning when sharks are most active.
- Never enter the water if there is a bleeding wound or when menstruating, as sharks have a very keen sense of smell and can easily detect blood.
- Don't wear shiny objects or bright-colored clothing in the water that may attract sharks.
- Avoid water which is dirty or contains sewage or water being used by fishermen, particularly if there are signs of bait fishes or feeding activity—seabirds diving for fish indicate such activity.
- Refrain from excess splashing, and do not allow pets in the water because their erratic behavior may attract sharks.
- Exercise caution in areas between the shore and sandbars or between sandbars because sharks may temporarily be trapped in these areas at low tide; many attacks occur in near-shore waters. Also, avoid swimming near steep drop-offs to greater depths because these are popular feeding zones for sharks.
- If swimming under water, keep the shark in sight—sharks seem to shy away from people who look directly at them! (The author of this book thinks he might blink!)
- Porpoises have only one fin on their back, whereas sharks have two; however, if you ever see fins in the water, don't wait to count fins. Instead, exit the water quickly and calmly.

Swimming Pools

When in the vicinity of a swimming pool, **young children should be constantly supervised, especially if they can't swim.** Drownings of young children have occurred in swimming pools, even in shallow water, because parents or chaperones have been distracted by friends or other children and were unaware that a child had disappeared below the surface of the water. Reports indicate that every day a child in Florida dies in a swimming pool. **It should be emphasized that neither adults nor children should ever swim alone** because, in the event of a severe injury or sudden illness, help from companions may be lifesaving. A course in lifesaving can be invaluable and is strongly recommended for those in their late teens and even for adults who are strong swimmers.

Contaminated Water

Finally, it should be remembered that lakes, fresh or brackish (somewhat salty) water, hot springs, or stagnant water, and even unmaintained swimming pools, may be contaminated with parasites that can cause serious illnesses and even death. This is particularly true in many foreign countries but may rarely occur in the United States. Therefore, one should not swim in water unless it is known to be clean and open for use by the public. Properly maintained and chlorinated swimming pools should be safe to use.

Safety in the Sun

Sunburns

Because sunburns can sometimes be severe and prolonged exposure to sunlight can cause skin cancers, including malignant melanomas, it is important for adults and children to avoid excessive exposure. **Proper precautions for skin protection from the sun should always be observed.** Sunscreens or tightly woven clothing and eliminating midday exposure to sunlight are very worthwhile protective measures. It is essential to educate parents and children about the hazards of excessive sunlight. **The New York State Department of Health has distributed valuable information on the**

importance of protecting the skin of children under the age of 13 years, as more than 90% of skin cancers are caused by sun exposure in childhood. The following are strongly recommended:

- Keep babies under 6 months of age out of the sun.
- Apply sunscreen with SPF 15 or higher to the entire body 30 minutes before sun exposure; choose waterproof or water-resistant products if the child is playing in the water. Apply sun screen about every 2 hours, but dry the skin first if wet or sweating.
- Limit the time children are exposed to the sun each day, and avoid skin exposure between 10 A.M. and 4 P.M., when the sun's ultraviolet rays (UV-A and UV-B) are strongest; cloudy or hazy days do not block most UV rays. These rays are not visible.
- Use wide-brimmed hats, long-sleeved shirts, long shorts or pants, and sunglasses (to protect the eyes and surrounding skin if you wish to limit exposure to sunlight).
- Keep babies and young children in the shade (e.g., under trees, umbrellas, or tents); strollers with hoods and canopies provide shade for babies and toddlers.
- Protect babies and young children from surfaces that can reflect the sun's damaging rays (e.g., sand, water, snow, and cement).
- Protect babies and young children from sun at high altitudes or in tropical climates where the sun's UV rays are especially strong.

Sun-burned or tanned skin is damaged skin, and the damage that adds up with each sunburn cannot be undone. **It is believed that most lifetime skin damage occurs before the age of 18 years.** It is always important for the parent to set a good example by following the recommendations they make to their children. Because some prescription and over-the-counter medications can increase skin sensitivity to sun exposure, it is prudent to consult with your physician or pharmacist regarding sun sensitivity that might be caused by any medication that you or your children are taking.

Malignant Melanoma

Finally, it may be lifesaving to learn to recognize the appearance of a malignant melanoma. The occurrence of this treacherous skin cancer has markedly increased during the past 40 years, possibly because of increased recreational sun exposure. Melanomas affect about 38,500 persons in the United States yearly and result in 8,000 deaths. **Adults of any age, and occasionally teenagers, may develop melanoma, and persons with light complexions, blond or red hair, blue eyes, and many freckles and moles are especially susceptible to developing this cancer.** However, heavily pigmented persons rarely develop melanomas. Heredity also plays a role in some individuals with this tumor, as about 10% have a family history of melanoma.

The ABCD rule provides the following clues that help identify melanomas:

A. Tumors are **Asymmetrical** (shapes are irregular, unlike most regular-shaped benign moles).

B. The **Border** is irregular (unlike the smooth edge of a benign mole).

C. The **Colors** of tumors may vary and may be partly black, brown, blue, white, and red (rather than one color in a benign mole).

D. The **Diameter** size of tumors is larger than the size of a pencil's eraser.

Sometimes melanomas become crusted and may bleed. Most melanomas occur on the back of men and on the lower legs of women; however, the individual should periodically check all areas of the skin. A spouse or friend should examine moles on the back. If there is the slightest concern that any characteristics of a melanoma appear, the individual should immediately consult a dermatologist. Those who have a large number of moles and those particularly susceptible to melanoma development should see a dermatologist annually.

Safety at Home

Fire

National fire facts indicate that 3 of 10 fires start in the kitchen and that cooking fires are the number one cause of home fires and home-fire injuries in the United States and Canada; **cigarettes or other smoking material are the number one cause of home fire deaths,** followed by heating equipment fires. **Candles are also responsible for many home fires** in the United States, and such fires are on the rise; it is urged that candles not be used in bedrooms.

Young children often have a curiosity about fire and are sometimes responsible for starting fires with matches or cigarette lighters. Some older children and teenagers who are emotionally upset or unstable, for a variety of reasons, may start a fire deliberately as an act of anger or defiance.

Smoke alarms in homes have been reported to cut the chance of dying in a fire by almost 50%; most states now require them in residential dwellings. **These alarms should be installed properly, and batteries should be changed yearly or whenever the alarm "chirps," indicating a low battery.** All members of the household should know the location of these smoke detectors and the sound of the alarm. For those with impaired hearing, louder alarm signals are available, and strobe (flashing) lights also can be used to alert these individuals that smoke is present. An escape plan should be practiced, and rapid exit through doors and windows should always be available. **Those who have exited a burning building are warned never to return until the fire department gives the OK.**

Young children must be prevented from burning themselves in fires or on hot stoves, hot kitchen utensils, uncovered hot radiators, or electric heaters. The Whirlpool Corporation has provided a number of very helpful tips:

1. **For Safer Cooking**
   - Always stay in the kitchen while cooking.
   - Turn pan handles away from the edge of the stove to avoid bumping them, which could cause spills of hot contents and possible burns.
   - Supervise children in the kitchen and teach them safety when cooking.
   - Wear short or close-fitting sleeves when cooking, and if wearing an apron, keep it securely tied.
   - Keep stove surfaces clean; grease buildups can catch fire.

2. **For Putting Out Cooking Fires**
   - Immediately call the fire department, dialing 911 for emergency services in most communities.
   - Smother a grease fire by covering it with a pan lid, and turn off the element or burner. Don't remove the lid until it cools. Smother other cooking fires with baking soda—don't use water.
   - Close the oven door, and turn off the heat to put out a fire in the oven.
   - Have the correct type of fire extinguisher nearby, and know how to use it.

Matches and lighters always must be kept out of the reach of children. Children should be taught by their parents about the danger of fire, and fire safety should be taught in school from preschool through high school.

Cigarettes must be properly discarded and never left burning. The possibility of falling asleep while smoking is extremely

hazardous. A mattress, sofa, or any upholstered furniture can easily become ignited by a cigarette that is not properly extinguished and can result in severe burns and fatalities. For those who smoke, it is especially wise to use fire-resistant materials wherever possible. Tossing a lit cigarette from the window while driving a vehicle can be extremely dangerous, as it can occasionally cause a devastating and deadly forest fire. Although a remote possibility, the tossed cigarette may re-enter the vehicle through an open rear window of the vehicle and cause a fire. This occurred recently when the lit cigarette ignited some flammable material in the rear of a car; the fire destroyed the car and severely burned the driver. **Warning: never throw a lit cigarette or cigar from a moving or even a stationary vehicle!**

Fires and candles must be extinguished if left unattended. Fireworks and pyrotechnics of any type should never be used by anyone except professionals, such as personnel of the fire department. Furthermore, the use of a blow torch to remove paint or solder pipes in a home can start a fire and should never be used except by a professionally qualified workman.

Finally, it is important to **dispose of rags or papers that contain oil or chemicals that may cause a fire by spontaneous combustion, that is without heating, and never keep gasoline in the house.**

Carbon Monoxide

As a safety precaution, carbon monoxide (CO) detectors should be installed in all homes and buildings that are heated by gas or oil or where any other fuel is burned. Carbon monoxide cannot be seen or smelled. If the CO detector alarm sounds, immediately turn off all gas appliances and other sources of combustion (e.g., furnace, water heaters, wood-burning stove). Get fresh air into the premises, and get professional assistance to fix the problem.

Some modern homes have pipes near the ground to exhaust fumes from heating equipment. **In regions where heavy snowfall occurs, it is important to have these exhaust pipes several feet above the ground to avoid the risk of snow blocking the exhaust of harmful fumes, including carbon monoxide. If exhaust pipes are close to the ground, it is imperative to prevent snow from blocking them.**

Gas Leaks and Fumes

As most are aware, natural gas used for home heating or for cooking gives a characteristic odor that is usually strongest on the floor, as natural gas does not rise. If a natural gas leak occurs that cannot be easily remedied, **never light a match or even use electrical equipment, including light switches, as this may cause a serious or fatal explosion. Promptly open windows to ventilate areas where you can smell gas. Always call your gas company immediately, and report that you smell gas.**

A very rare but potentially serious hazard is the occurrence of an explosion while filling the tank of a vehicle with gasoline. **Gasoline fumes** can be ignited with a spark generated by static electricity. Therefore, no one should walk about near the area of refueling to avoid generating a spark. If the person refueling does not move about and remains grounded by first touching a metal object, the hazard of an explosion should be prevented.

Knives and Sharp Instruments

Knives and sharp instruments should be kept from the grasp of children. **Any deep wound** (e.g., from a knife, nail, rake, or any sharp object) **requires immediate medical attention**, and sometimes an injection to prevent tetanus ("lock jaw") is indicated, particularly if the wound is contaminated with dirt.

Window Bars and Safety Gates

It is extremely important that open windows are not accessible to young children. Window bars to prevent fatal falls of young children are especially helpful. Safety gates at the top of staircases can prevent young children from falling down the stairs.

Tools and Machinery

Operating tractors, mowers, chain saws, and other commonplace household tools and machinery can be hazardous, especially if using medications that interfere with alertness or judgment. **Children, especially, should be kept away from running machinery.** It is reported that each year nearly 10,000 children and teenagers 15 years old or younger are injured by lawn mowers.

Pistols and Guns

Pistols and **guns** pose a very real risk; **they must never be left loaded. Above all, they should always be locked in a secure location, accessible only to a responsible owner.** Guns and pistols should *never* be left loaded and accessible to anyone except the owner. Innumerable tragedies have occurred because some young child or teenager handled a loaded firearm that then discharged and injured or killed someone nearby. If all firearms were locked in a secure location and not accessible, it is likely that the number of these tragedies would plummet. Furthermore, the number of senseless random shootings that have occurred periodically in high schools in the United States would probably markedly decrease. Informing children and teenagers about the dangers of handling pistols and guns and keeping firearms inaccessible should be a major concern of all parents. It may be difficult, if not impossible, to identify older children and teenagers who might become violent and seriously injure others; however, parents and teachers should work together and report any manifestations of deep depression, anger, violent fantasies, or severe emotional behavior by teenagers that may require medical consultation and treatment.

Electric Shock

Children must be cautioned about the dangers of electrical shock from wall and bulb sockets and electric appliances. Extension cords may also be faulty and responsible for shocks or fire. **Caution should be observed particularly when electrical appliances are used, especially in bathrooms, and they must never be used in wet bathtubs.**

Safe Food Preparation

Many travelers to foreign countries, especially remote regions, are aware that to prevent infections they should avoid drinking un-bottled or unpasteurized fluids and eating uncooked foods, salads, and fruits. It is wise to use bottled water, even when brushing teeth. However, it is also essential to mention and stress the importance of cleanliness during food preparation in everyday life in the United States.

With regard to food preparation, you should always remember, "Food that is safe from harmful bacteria, viruses, parasites, and chemical contaminants is vital for healthful eating." **Food-borne illness can result from food containing bacteria (e.g., Salmonella, Listeria, Campylobacter, E. coli, Shigella, Staphylococcus, or Clostridium), toxins (substances released from bacteria), viruses (e.g., Norwalk "24-hour stomach bug" or Norwalk-like viruses), parasites (e.g., amoebae), and chemical contaminants. These germs or chemicals may cause vomiting, diarrhea, abdominal pains, fever, and flu-like symptoms.** Young children, older persons, pregnant women, and those with chronic or immunodeficient diseases are particularly at risk for contracting these illnesses.

To avoid food-borne disease, you should not drink unpasteurized milk (or products made from unpasteurized milk) or unpasteurized juices. Pregnant women should particularly avoid foods that are most likely to be contaminated with Listeria, as infection with this bacteria can cause spontaneous abortion and stillbirth. The most likely contaminated foods include milk and milk products (especially soft cheeses such as feta, Brie, Camembert, blue-veined cheeses, and Mexican style cheeses) that are unpasteurized. It is risky to eat hot dogs and luncheon or deli meats, especially during pregnancy, unless they are reheated until steaming hot. Unpasteurized pâté and meat spreads should be avoided (canned pâté and meat spreads that don't require refrigeration are safe). It is, of course, important to avoid using foods or drinks that may possibly be contaminated, if seals are not intact. It is always risky to eat raw or undercooked food (meat, poultry, eggs, fish, and shellfish). Properly washing hands, food, utensils, cutting boards, and any equipment used in preparing food is essential to prevent transmission of germs.

To warn those who may be adventurous and willing to abandon precautions when eating raw food, the following true story is worth recounting:

Case Report

P.D., a distinguished medical doctor, had returned from a vacation in Europe. He began to experience abdominal pains and elevations of his temperature up to 103°F. He became progressively debilitated, a condition that greatly concerned his physicians, as no obvious cause was evident. A CAT scan (X-ray) of his abdomen revealed what appeared to be cysts in his liver.

Consultation with Dr. Jonathan LaPook, an outstanding specialist in stomach, intestinal, and liver disease, was arranged. After reviewing the X-rays, Dr. LaPook determined that the cysts might be caused by a rare parasite called Fasciola Hepatica. This astute specialist then asked, "Did you eat any raw watercress while you were in Europe?" P.D. answered that while he and his wife were touring in Ireland, they picked and ate a considerable amount of watercress without washing it. The danger of not thoroughly washing watercress growing in the fields is that sheep infected with Fasciola Hepatica may urinate on the watercress and contaminate it with this parasite.

The next step was to establish the suspected diagnosis, as only a specific treatment can eradicate this parasitic infection. The tenacity of Dr. LaPook paid off because although the diagnostic blood test was not available in the United States, the test could be done by a physician in Paris; a specimen of blood was immediately sent to him. The diagnosis was established, and appropriate treatment was begun. The patient recovered fully; however, he has totally lost his taste for watercress, even in the finest restaurants!

Guidelines for safe food preparation are available free of charge from the U.S. Department of Health and Human Services or Department of Agriculture. For everyone, the following is recommended:

1. Wash hands with warm soapy water for at least 20 seconds before handling food, utensils, and cutting boards and after handling or preparing food. Discard cutting boards with grooves that cannot be cleaned adequately. Wash fruits and vegetables and remove surface dirt. Always wash hands after using the toilet or after changing diapers or handling pets. (Exit public restrooms by using a paper towel or glove or your jacket or coat to open a door and prevent contaminating your hand.) Hand washing is extremely important in preventing or minimizing transmission of a variety of viruses that cause illness, including the common cold. Whenever possible, avoid touching your nose, eyes, or mouth with unwashed hands.

2. Keep raw food away from contact with other food surfaces, utensils, or serving plates prevents cross-contamination from one food to another. Refrigerate and store raw food (meat, poultry, fish, and shellfish) in containers so that their juices don't come in contact with other foods. Never thaw frozen meat, poultry, fish, or shellfish at room temperature; thaw in the refrigerator and then remove for food preparation.

3. Cook uncooked meat and poultry to safe temperatures ranging from 140°F to 180°F. If using a microwave, stir or turn food to make sure that it is thoroughly cooked. Cooking vegetables in a microwave can destroy most of the healthful chemicals (antioxidants) that may protect against some kinds of heart disease, cancers, and infections. However, steaming vegetables causes very little loss of these beneficial chemicals. Reheat sauces, soups, and gravies to a boil, and reheat leftovers thoroughly to 165°F. Cook eggs until the whites or yokes are firm.

4. Refrigerate (at 40°F) or freeze (at 0°F) perishable foods promptly. Freeze fresh meat, poultry, fish, and shellfish that will not be used within a few days.

5. Follow instructions on food labels.

6. Keep hot foods at 140°F or above and cold foods at 40°F or below to prevent bacterial growth, which can occur rapidly between these temperatures (the "danger zone").

7. Discard food that may not have been prepared or stored safely—"When in doubt, throw it out." The old saying "keep it hot or keep it cold or don't keep it" is worth remembering.

8. Despite the pleasure of dining outdoors at a restaurant or picnic, sometimes food may become contaminated by germ-carrying flies or other insects. Open buffets may also become contaminated by handling utensils and food with unwashed hands. It is important to keep food covered when it is not being eaten, as contamination may cause serious disease.

9. Food should not come directly in contact with a desk or table-top that has not been cleaned. Unclean surfaces usually contain bacteria that may contaminate food and cause illness.

10. Finally, even the safest food preparation and cooking cannot destroy certain toxins (poisons) that may be present in some marine life. Moray eels, blue-ringed octopus, puffer fish, tropical coral reef fish, and parrot fish should never be eaten, as they may contain toxins that can cause serious illness and occasionally death. Severe reactions to toxins also have been reported after eating barracuda, snapper, jack, and grouper. Those who have experienced a severe illness after eating any of these fish should especially avoid eating these fish in the future, as a second reaction may be more severe and possibly life-threatening.

For more information, contact the USDA's Meat and Poultry Hotline, 1-800-535-4555, or the FDA's Food Information Line, 1-888-723-3366. Another excellent Web resource is Fight Bac, the Partnership for Food Safety Education (http://www.fightbac.org).

Safety of Children

Toy Safety

Most parents or guardians recognize toy safety as an extremely important concern for young children. The Child Safety Protection Act requires toy manufacturers to place warning labels on toys containing small parts that may be ingested by children under 3 years of age and cause airway obstruction, choking, and sometimes death. **Parents should carefully examine toys to make sure that there are no small objects (e.g., balls, marbles, parts of stuffed animals, or uninflated balloons) that may be ingested and cause choking with an inability to breathe. If there is evidence of sudden**

airway obstruction, the child should be immediately held in a position with face looking downward. It may then be possible to dislodge an obstructing object by delivering several moderate blows to the back between the shoulder blades. If this doesn't relieve the obstruction, call 911 or rush the child to an emergency room if one is nearby. Airway obstruction is the leading cause of toy death.

Tragic deaths occur in young children when hard candy is aspirated (breathed in) and obstructs the airway. Round balls of candy the size of a large grape are particularly hazardous. However, any hard candy can be aspirated. Therefore, any hard candy should be broken up before it is given to a young child. One emergency room pediatrician reported that 60% of choking cases he sees in the emergency room result from eating grapes, peanuts, or hot dogs, but another 20% involve eating hard candy. About 90% of choking cases occur in children under 5 years of age.

It is essential and may be lifesaving to alert the public constantly to the potential serious risks of choking in young children caused by certain foods or candy or by small play objects that may obstruct the airway.

With regards to airway obstruction, it **is extremely important to place a baby or infant** (up to 3 years of age) **on their back with the head facing up when sleeping.** If placed on the stomach with the head facing down, the airway may become obstructed by the mattress, pillow, or covers and may cause suffocation and death.

The following precautions have been recommended for infants and young children:

- Avoid access to objects that can be ingested.
- Avoid toys with sharp points or edges.
- Discard plastic wrappers and bags, as they may cause suffocation if the child places these over the head. Explain the dangers

of placing a plastic bag over the head to children who are old enough to understand the danger of suffocation.

- Do not fire caps in toy guns close to the ears because the noise may impair hearing.
- Avoid toys that shoot small objects, as they may injure someone's eye.
- Avoid toys with strings or cords, as the latter may become wrapped around a child's neck and cause strangulation.
- Do not hang toys over a crib or play pen because the infant may become entangled in them. Do not place a crib or play pen near any cords (e.g., venetian blind cords) to prevent possible entanglement.
- Use a toy box that has ventilation holes. Do not use boxes or pieces of furniture for storing toys, as a child might become trapped without adequate air. Warn children to never get into the trunk of a car or a discarded refrigerator because of the danger of being trapped. Keep a car trunk locked at all times, and dispose of old refrigerators that are not being used; secure or remove the door.
- Be careful when selecting electrical toys with heating elements that may cause burns.

Clothing Safety

Avoid wearing jackets with **long cords** or **long scarves** that may become entangled on exiting a vehicle or on a rope tow or chairlift at a ski area because they may cause a person to be dragged or strangled and severely injured or killed. Avoid loose **shoe laces** that may be caught in escalators or cause children to trip and injure themselves.

Pedophiles

It is important for every child to be warned to avoid contact with strangers. Parents should explain the risks of being abducted and sexually assaulted. *Pedophilia* **(i.e., sexual perversion in which**

children are the sexual object and desire of an adult) is a serious problem in the United States where 500,000 sex offenders are registered; they frequently reside in poor areas. Most who prey on children and other sex offenders have never been arrested. Pedophiles are psychopaths (those without a conscience) who sexually molest children and sometimes kill them. It must be recognized that these individuals cannot be reformed, and if they return to society after imprisonment, they pose a constant threat for repeating sexual molestation of a child. Parents must have a vigilant eye and supervise young children as much as possible. *Never* **leave children with anyone you can't trust. If you are employing a babysitter, be sure that they have provided excellent references that are reliable. Beware of strangers or neighbors who become overly interested in children.** Sometimes they may offer marijuana or alcohol to children if parents are not present.

If a stranger stops their car and tries to grab a child by the arm and coax him or her into the car, the child should quickly swing their arm over their head to release the adult's grip. Children should immediately start yelling for help and run away as fast as possible to find a safe location where adults are present.

Children and adults are more likely to be sexually assaulted or abused by family members or friends than strangers. It is reported that in the United States domestic violence is the main cause of injury to females between the ages of 15 and 44 years old. Any physical abuse should be reported immediately to the police.

Doors should always be locked at night, and it is wise for parents to leave their bedroom door slightly open so that they might be able to hear an intruder enter the house through a door or window. An alarm system to detect an intruder is especially desirable. Unfortunately, many sex offenders are lost to follow-up after release from prison. It would be very helpful if all sex and pedophile offenders were forced to wear an electronic bracelet or anklet that would constantly keep these predators under close surveillance.

It is strongly recommended that the public become aware of some of the Internet websites supplying the names and locations of pedophiles and other sex offenders. Check the following websites: www.nationalalertregistry.com and www.childsafenet.org.

It is of paramount importance that anyone caring for young children be made aware of this information and recommendations. It is vital that when parents are not at home they leave telephone numbers and locations where they can be reached immediately in case of any emergency involving a baby or child.

Safety of Older People

Falls

Special efforts should be made to protect persons 65 years or older from falling and incurring severe head injuries and fractures. About one third of older persons fall each year, although many of these falls can be prevented. Hip fractures are particularly common and severe in older persons, especially for those with osteoporosis (bone thinning).

- **With aging, about 30% of older individuals have an excessive drop in blood pressure on standing,** which can cause dizziness and fainting. Sedatives, sleeping and heart medications, anticonvulsants, antidepressants, and some antihypertensive drugs also may cause a drop in blood pressure on standing, in addition to weakness, unsteadiness, and sometimes fainting that can result in a fall.
- **Inadequate daily consumption of fluid can cause dehydra-**

tion, which may play a role in a diminished blood pressure. It is recommended that six to eight glasses of fluid be consumed daily by most individuals of normal height and weight. Occasionally, a physician may recommend extra salt in the diet for those with low blood pressures.

- **Visual impairment, diminished muscle strength, and decreased balance when walking may be responsible for falls. Provide adequate lighting in dark areas.**
- **Removal of unstable "throw" rugs, avoidance of slippery floors and sidewalks, safer foot wear, nonslip bath mats, night lighting, and stair rails are strongly recommended. Cover slippery areas with material that will not move.**
- **Toys should be removed from the floor, as they may cause persons to trip, and special caution should be observed when using stairs or ladders.**
- **Working with a therapist or exercise group to improve muscle strength and minimize unsteady walking may be very helpful.** Walking slowly and carefully with a wider base (feet farther apart) and wearing low-heeled shoes can be helpful; the use of a cane or walker may also be necessary.
- **Older persons should always be seated when they are putting on pants, socks, or stockings; this will prevent falls that can easily occur if individuals are standing.**
- **Underpants with hip padding may help reduce hip injuries.**
- **Individuals, especially older persons, can minimize the possibility of twisting an ankle and/or falling if they are careful to avoid stepping on depressions or elevations in sidewalks or when crossing streets.** Remember whenever walking, "Watch Your Step!"
- **Physicians should review all medications and reduce some if indicated.** It was recently reported that, each year, the average U.S. senior citizen fills prescriptions for about eight different medications. Seniors frequently use a number of different pharmacies and see a number of different doctors who may not be

aware of all the medications being used. To avoid serious drug reactions and dangerous drug interactions, it is extremely important to keep doctors informed of all medications and any "health supplements" being consumed. Even over-the-counter sleeping medications (especially if taken in excess) may cause some confusion and instability that can cause an older or frail person to fall and be severely injured. Remaining seated on the side of the bed for a minute or two may permit adequate circulation to the brain before standing. It is also wise to block a stairway and ensure adequate illumination to minimize the possibility of a serious fall.

According to the Mayo Clinic, weakened muscles are the most important cause of falls in older adults and the main cause for falls and fall-related deaths in those over 65 years of age. Persons begin losing muscle strength at 40 years of age, and this accelerates after age 75. This age-related decrease in muscle size and loss of muscle strength is called sarcopenia. Dr. Nair at the Mayo Clinic (a leading center for understanding the cause and cure of sarcopenia) says that flexing and stretching, weight lifting, and aerobic exercise (e.g., walking, running, swimming) are three important exercises for maintaining muscle strength. Mayo Clinic researchers indicate that strong muscles "prevent chronic illness, weight gain, general frailty, and even mental decline," and that a program to improve muscle strength can be started at any age. They point out four main ways of preventing falls:

1. Exercise regularly.
2. Make your home safe (about half of all falls occur in the home)—use nonslip mats in bath tubs and showers, install grab bars, remove small rugs that can cause tripping, use bright lights, install hand rails in all staircases.
3. Review all medications with your doctor annually.
4. Have your vision checked, since poor vision can cause falls.

It is *extremely* important for persons taking blood thinners to avoid a head injury, since often a blow to the head may cause fatal bleeding in the brain in these individuals.

- **Fear of falling is very common in older persons and may cause them to decrease their mobility and thus, further decrease muscle strength and agility.** According to Professor J. Howland of Boston University, fear of falling may cause significant depression, which can lead to use of sedatives and increased alcohol consumption and thereby enhance the likelihood of falling. The older population must receive proper consultation and guidance that can minimize the chance of injuries from falling. Installing hand rails in appropriate locations and the use of assisted mobility devices ("walkers" of various types) can often prevent falling and serious injuries.

Sensitivity to Heat and Cold

Older persons are more vulnerable to excessive heat or cold than most younger persons. Therefore, adequate air conditioning or heating is essential for their safety. Because persons with high blood pressure appear more susceptible to heart attacks in cold weather, it is especially important for these persons to wear warm clothes when indicated and to avoid very cold weather.

Living Alone

It is extremely important that older persons, who live or may at times be left alone, have an electronic alarm device attached to their clothing or hanging from their neck. In case of an emergency, activation of the alarm will immediately summon help. Possessing such an alarm also provides a welcome sense of security and peace of mind to older persons who may be alone.

Environmental Hazards

Poisonings

Medicines, alcohol, poisons, and chemicals of any type must be secured or out of the reach of children. Also, it is especially important to prevent children from eating or chewing wild-growing berries, mushrooms, leaves, or seeds that may contain naturally occurring poisons (e.g., the deadly poison ricin occurs in bean-like seeds of the castor plant). The U.S. Poison Center can be contacted, if necessary, by telephone at 1-800-222-1222 or in New York at 1-212-POISONS.

Mercury

Excess mercury in some fish has already been mentioned; contaminated fish are the most likely source of mercury poisoning. Because mercury is a liquid that cannot be broken down and evaporates quickly, incineration of any product containing mercury will cause it to be released into the air and spread by wind until it settles on the earth or water. Mercury poisoning can cause damage of the brain and nerves with personality changes, mental deterioration, neurological manifestations, and even death if poisoning is severe.

Women who may become pregnant or are nursing and children must be careful about how much and what type of fish they eat. It is recommended that no more than 3 to 6 ounces of tuna be consumed per week. *Consumer Reports* **recommends that children and pregnant women avoid eating Albacore tuna because it usually has higher levels of mercury.** King mackerel, shark, swordfish, and tilefish may also have high levels of mercury. Other fish and shellfish usually have low levels of mercury, but your regional or state

environmental protection agency can give you additional information about the safety of eating fish in your area. Currently, there is
an effort to discontinue use of mercury-containing devices to reduce the hazards of contamination. Products containing mercury,
including some batteries used for toys, hearing aids, and watches,
should never be incinerated but should be disposed of in a landfill.
If you are concerned about the amount of mercury in your body, a
blood test can easily be performed.

Lead

It is a misconception that lead poisoning affects only the poor living in inner-city neighborhoods where buildings are often deteriorating. Anyone can be exposed to paint dust containing lead
during renovations of older homes. Young children are at special
risk for developing lead poisoning since they crawl and play on the
floor and ground where they can easily ingest or inhale paint dust
or chips that contain lead. **Absorption of lead through the lungs or
stomach can cause toxic levels, particularly in young children, but
also in others who are repeatedly exposed to lead. Eating from
lead-glazed dishes (more commonly found in tableware made in
South America or Mexico), taking certain medicines used in
India, using water boiled in leaded pots and pans, and continually
using some foreign cosmetics and certain foreign cold medications, spices, and foods can ultimately cause lead poisoning.** Exposure to a variety of other sources of lead (e.g., fumes from leaded
gasoline or from soldering lead, battery manufacturing, or recy-
cling plants and other lead industries) may be encountered, but
unless exposure to lead is repeated and prolonged, the chance of
lead poisoning is very unlikely. Pencils contain graphite for writing and not lead; however, some toys may contain lead. The New
York City Department of Health and Mental Hygiene recommends taking special precautions if your job or hobby (construc-
tion, bridge maintenance, home renovation and repair, furniture
refinishing, automotive and electronic repair, making stained glass

or pottery, and bullet dust from target practice at a firing range) involves exposure to lead. Don't bring work clothes or shoes into the house if your job or hobby exposes you to lead.

Excess amounts of lead in the body can damage many organs, especially the brain, nerves, kidneys, and blood cells. Common symptoms of lead poisoning include fatigue, depression, kidney and heart failure, constipation, severe abdominal pain, vomiting, high blood pressure, wrist and foot weakness, lowered IQ, anemia, decreased appetite, convulsions, and rarely death.

If there is any concern about lead exposure or poisoning, consult a physician. A blood test can detect elevations of lead, and it is critical to test all children at ages 1 and 2 years for elevated lead in their blood. Effective treatment is available for removing lead from the body.

Homes may be checked for lead, and experts can remove leaded paint. Professional advice on ways to reduce exposure to lead can be obtained. It is crucial to reduce or avoid contact with painted interior and exterior walls, doors, windows, and paint dust and soil around houses built before 1978. In New York City, peeling and chipping paint and household dust containing lead are reportedly the main source of children's exposure. It is important to clean floors and windowsills frequently with a wet mop or wet cloth, as lead dust is often found in these places. Also, wash children's hands, toys, pacifiers, and bottles frequently to remove lead dust.

It is recommended that tap water obtained from lead pipes in old houses be run for 60 seconds before using it for drinking or cooking if water has not been run for several hours. It is wise to test water for lead safety particularly in old houses or buildings built before 1960; this can be done by government agencies. The Environmental Protection Agency is playing a major role in reducing the hazards of lead exposure. It is advised that healthcare providers annually assess all children 6 months to 6 years of age for risk of lead exposure and provide their families with education about preventing lead poisoning.

Asbestos

Asbestos fiber has been used for strengthening cement and plastics, insulating pipes, fireproofing, and sound absorption, and it has been especially used in the shipbuilding and automotive industries. **It is found in many old homes where it has been used for furnace and pipe insulation, in shingles, in floor tiles, and in acoustical material.**

The danger of asbestos is that particles of asbestos, usually too small to see, may become airborne after cutting, sanding, during building renovations, and in attempts to remove it. **Therefore, it is extremely important to avoid disturbing any asbestos-containing material and to engage the help of professionals who are knowledgeable in properly handling asbestos to minimize or eliminate the risk of exposure to this potentially deadly substance.** Sometimes sealing off asbestos may be preferable to removing it, but this requires the advice of an expert.

Asbestos dust can be inhaled or swallowed and can cause (1) lung cancer and other cancers of the respiratory and gastrointestinal tracts and the kidney, (2) mesothelioma (a malignant tumor of the tissues lining the chest and abdomen), and (3) asbestosis (a scarring of lung tissue making it difficult to breathe). Symptoms of these diseases, which are usually fatal, may occur 10 to 40 years after the onset of exposure to asbestos particles. The risk of developing lung cancer in smokers is greatly increased with prolonged inhalation of asbestos dust. **Anyone exposed to asbestos dust should definitely not smoke.** Chronic asbestos exposure on the job is especially hazardous and requires rigid precautions to prevent inhalation or ingestion of these potentially lethal particles. Those who must work with asbestos should make certain that their bodies, shoes, and clothes do not contain asbestos dust that could contaminate their family and others.

Individuals who may have been exposed to asbestos dust should inform their doctor. A chronic cough (especially if sputum contains blood), shortness of breath, prolonged hoarseness, pain in the chest or abdomen, difficulty swallowing, or unexpected weight loss may be a consequence of disease caused by asbestos exposure. Asbestos can be measured in the urine and in material obtained from the lungs. Special chest X-rays may be indicated.

The U.S. Environmental Protection Agency recommends that "it is best to leave undamaged asbestos material alone if it is not likely to be disturbed." However, it should be appreciated that gradual deterioration of ceilings containing asbestos tiles may release significant amounts of asbestos particles into the air. Furthermore, it may be difficult or impossible to avoid disturbing damaged and deteriorating floor and wall surfaces containing asbestos.

Make certain that you give top priority to protecting your family and yourself from possible exposure to asbestos dust and seek the consultation and advice of an expert in handling asbestos.

Additional information about asbestos is available from the U.S. Department of Health and Human Services and local and state health agencies.

Arsenic

Because ingesting toxic amounts of arsenic may cause lung or kidney cancer, there has been concern about young children coming in contact with potentially dangerous levels of arsenic in pressure-treated wood in playgrounds. Arsenic is used to make wood last longer and to prevent deterioration caused by bugs and fungi.

Children may get some of this arsenic on their hands and fingers and transmit it to their mouths. Recently, arsenic-treated wood has been banned, and lumber firms have discontinued producing it. Older wood can be sealed to eliminate arsenic contamination.

Mold/Fungi

Exposure to high concentrations of mold (fungus) in the air may occasionally cause irritation of the lungs and pneumonia, allergic asthma, or infection in some susceptible persons. However, although mold-related illness appears to be very rare, it is important to remove mold and to prevent or remedy water damage and dampness, which can result in mold growth within buildings. Recently, there has been excessive and unjustified concern about the health risks posed by exposure to mold. As a result, lawsuits have increased dramatically with claims that repair of water damage and water leaks were improperly delayed and resulted in mold-related symptoms.

Ingestion of toadstools, which are molds, can cause severe illness or death. It is imperative that children be warned about the danger of eating any wild-growing substance that may be poisonous and fatal if consumed. **Very young children must, of course, be constantly watched to prevent access to any poisonous substance.**

Weather-Related Hazards

Lightning

For those living in houses in rural areas, it is prudent to have lightning rods for protection during severe electrical storms. Although some are skeptical regarding the need for lightning rods, fire department personnel will readily confirm the value of this protection. It is important to understand and respect the danger of electrocution from lightning during a severe thunderstorm. **The safest precaution is to remain in a closed house or a closed car** (rubber tires prevent grounding and prohibit damage from lightning). If one is outdoors and cannot reach a house or car, **avoid refuge near trees, telephone poles, hilltops, hedges, or riverbanks. No one should remain in a swimming pool or other water.** To take refuge in a cave, under a roadway bridge, or in a ditch is quite safe. Even lying on the ground in a curled up position with hands close together is recommended as relatively safe. **It is, however, dangerous to remain in a car if a severe hurricane or tornado is developing nearby.** One should exit the car immediately and enter a building or seek a low-lying area or ditch. One freak electrocution occurred recently in New York City. The car in which two young adults were riding stalled in a flash flood. During the storm, lightning struck a nearby utility pole, causing a 2,400 volt power line to fall into the water. Tragically, the occupants of the car were not aware that the water carried a powerful electrical charge, and both were electrocuted when they exited the car and stepped into the water.

Hurricanes/Floods

Hurricanes are high winds with speeds over 74 mph; speeds may reach 200 mph or more. They usually move at a rate of about 10 mph and last for 1 to 30 days. Hurricanes, which arise over the ocean as a tropical storm, occur in United States costal areas most often in September but they may occur from June 1st through December 1st.

Warm water will intensify the severity of a hurricane. A hurricane (named Katrina) in late August 2005 reached a wind speed of 175 mph (the top category 5 storm) as it passed over the Gulf of Mexico where the surface water temperature was 90° F, that is, hotter than the air temperature. When it struck the coasts of Mississippi and Louisiana, the wind had decreased to 145 mph (category 4);

however, the destruction was extreme in parts of Mississippi and Louisiana but also affected parts of Alabama and Florida. A surge of water which struck parts of the coast of Mississippi was reported to be 25 feet high. The greatest damage and death occurred in New Orleans because of flooding when water broke through levees and submerged and isolated 80% of the city. Unfortunately, New Orleans is below sea level, and destruction of some of the levees by the hurricane permitted enormous amounts of water from Lake Pontchartrain to flow freely into New Orleans and flood the city. Sadly, about one thousand perished in this disaster.

In September 1938, a category 3 hurricane suddenly struck the eastern end of Long Island and then moved North through parts of Rhode Island, where it caused extensive flooding. Six hundred lives were lost, and property damage was enormous. Weather forecasters state that the cool ocean temperature makes it impossible for a category 5 hurricane to reach Long Island, and that a category 4 is extremely unlikely. However, category 3 hurricanes and lesser hurricanes may periodically strike the East Coast and cause extensive damage. However, with the ability to warn residents of an approaching hurricane, loss of life should be minimal—the key is for those in harm's way to evacuate areas before the hurricane reaches land.

The cause of these violent storms is not known. Hurricanes are frequently accompanied by torrential rains, flash floods, and inland flooding, which may extend 20 miles inland. **Flooding is responsible for most deaths. Especially dangerous and damaging is a hurricane surge that creates a dome of ocean water that may reach a height of 25 feet and extend 50 to 100 miles wide and cause devastating damage to coastal regions of the United States.** After initial severe hurricane winds, which rotate as a spiral, the eye in the center of the storm, which may be 20 to 30 miles wide with little or no wind, may pass over an area giving the impression that the hurricane is over. Those unfamiliar with hurricanes may leave a safe area and venture outside only to be killed by the return of severe wind as the eye passes by.

Injury and death can result from trauma caused by collapsing buildings or flying debris, which may inflict severe wounds and even impale an individual. However, most deaths result from injuries caused by inland flooding and drowning. A particularly serious hazard can be caused by a high-voltage power line that has been severed by a fallen tree; this exposed current can cause a fire, but as mentioned previously, it also can electrify the water it contacts and generate a current that can electrocute any one stepping into the water. It is crucial for those leaving or re-entering a dwelling in a flooded area to be certain that there are no high-voltage wires in contact with any water that must be crossed.

If you live in a hurricane zone, find out whether your home meets the building code requirements for protection from high winds. The roof may be particularly vulnerable to damage. Hurricanes can easily destroy poorly constructed buildings and mobile homes. It is recommended that windows and glass doors be protected by storm shutters or 5/8-inch plywood. Garage doors frequently need to be reinforced, and outside furniture and any objects that can be airborne and become dangerous flying missiles should be placed indoors when possible.

It is usually possible for meteorologists to predict the path of a hurricane and anticipate the time of arrival and the speed of the wind. **If you are told to evacuate an area, it is wise to turn off all utilities, fill your car with gas, and use designated evacuation routes to the nearest possible safe location.** Complacency and delayed action could result in needless injury or loss of life. It is important to consider how best to transport persons in a household. Older persons, those who are handicapped, and those who are ill will need assistance. Prepare a separate plan to evacuate pets because most public shelters do not accept pets. The safest internal rooms are those with no windows or external doors. In high rise buildings, stay below the 10th floor and above any floors at risk for flooding.

It has been reported that decreased barometric (atmospheric) pressure associated with hurricanes may hasten the onset of labor in some pregnant women. Although the evidence for this claim has not been scientifically established, it is especially important for pregnant women who are near the time of delivery to stay in close contact with their obstetrician and to follow evacuation instructions.

Certain rules should be observed. For example, **never drive across a flooded road.** Moving water can exert very strong pressure on a person or a car. The large size of a sport utility vehicle and its large tires can make it especially buoyant and just as prone to being swept away as other cars. **Two feet of moving water can carry away most cars. If your car stalls in a flooded area and the water is rising, abandon the vehicle immediately. Do not try to walk across a flooded area greater than knee deep. If you are in a building and the water is rising, move to a higher floor and wait for help. Never try to swim to safety.**

It is strongly recommended to have the following disaster supplies stored together in a convenient location:

- Several flashlights with extra batteries (flashlights are available that do not need battery replacement and are shock and water-proof)
- A portable battery-operated radio with extra batteries
- A first-aid kit and essential medications
- Emergency food with a manual can opener and drinking water that is adequate for several days (do not drink tap water until notified it is safe)
- Cash in small denominations and credit cards

- Shoes or sneakers and change of clothing
- Copies of all important papers
- A fully charged cellular phone

Beware of downed or loose power lines and report these whenever possible. Above all, keep in frequent contact with weather reports, and follow evacuation instructions.

Tornadoes

A tornado is a violent, whirling wind that usually appears as a dark funnel that extends from heavy clouds in the sky to the ground. The funnel twists, rises, and falls and moves at a rate of 20 to 40 mph. Some may occur over water. Occasionally, a tornado may be produced by a hurricane, but the cause of this treacherous, whirling wind, that may reach a speed of 200 to 300 mph is not known. At the bottom of the funnel-shaped tornado is extremely low air pressure that causes a strong updraft that acts like a giant vacuum. Tornadoes are frequently associated with severe thunderstorms and heavy rain. They usually occur in the spring and in the late afternoon or early evening, but they may occur any time of the year. In the United States, tornadoes occur most commonly on the Great Plains—often called "Tornado Alley." **Some have described the following just before the arrival of a tornado:**

- A greenish or greenish-black color in the sky
- Hail
- A very quiet period after a thunderstorm
- Clouds moving very fast, especially if rotating
- A sound like a waterfall or rushing air initially and then a roar as it comes closer
- Debris dropping from the sky
- A funnel-shaped cloud or debris, branches, or leaves being pulled upward, even if no funnel is visible

It has been said that "if you see a tornado not moving to the right or left, it may be moving toward you."

It is important to plan several different locations where members of a family should go rapidly in the event of an approaching tornado. The following locations have been recommended for safety during a tornado:

- Storm shelter designed for placement in the ground
- Basement of a building, where staying under a sturdy table or under stairs will provide further protection from crumbling walls and falling debris
- Small, windowless interior rooms on the 1st floor, for example, a closet or bathroom

The more walls between you and the tornado, the better. Placing a trash can over the head may prevent head injuries.

Families should practice tornado drills so that everyone will know what to do and where to go to minimize the chance of injury when a tornado strikes.

The same disaster supplies recommended during a hurricane also should be available during a tornado. **Auditoriums and gyms in schools should be vacated, and children and adults should go to interior rooms and halls on lower floors but avoid halls opening to the outside and follow directions from teachers and adults.**

Always leave a car and seek shelter. Most deaths occur in cars and mobile homes. In the event of a tornado, it is important for family members to be prepared to act promptly to protect themselves from an approaching tornado.

Earthquakes/Tsunamis

Earthquakes vary from slight tremors to violent vibrations of the earth's surfaces caused by a sudden release of force from a fracture of large blocks of rocks with a shifting of the earth's crust or rocky outer shell. Usually, minor earthquakes accompany volcanic eruptions. They usually last for a few minutes, but aftershocks may continue for days or weeks. The severity of an earthquake can be measured on the Richter scale (1 being the mildest and 7 being a major quake; rarely do the most severe exceed 8).

Earthquakes almost never directly kill; injuries and death result from falling objects, collapsing buildings, bridges, overpasses, dams, and other structures, landslides, spills of hazardous chemicals, and fires resulting from broken gas and power lines. The deadliest natural disaster in the United States occurred in 1906 in San Francisco when an earthquake and accompanying fire killed about 6,000 people. Large earthquakes beneath the ocean floor can create huge destructive waves called **tsunamis,** which may travel up to 600 or more mph below the surface of the ocean with little disturbance of the ocean surface and little effect on ships and small boats. However, when a tsunami reaches shallow water in coastal regions, a gigantic wave, sometimes over 200 feet high, suddenly develops and often drowns thousands of individuals in coastal and adjacent areas. These waves are not only extremely dangerous but they are deceptive because, after the devastation of this initial wave, there may be a rapid water withdrawal from the coast. This may suggest the end of the tsunami; however, subsequent huge waves may rapidly reoccur and drown individuals who have returned to the coast.

The tsunami does not usually engulf and kill individuals a mile or more from the coast or those on high ground at elevations 100 or more feet above sea level. Unfortunately, scientists are unable to predict when and where a tsunami will strike. Without any accurate warning system, these "killer" waves continue to be extremely destructive, often causing thousands of deaths. In 2004, the tsunami, traveling at a rate of about 500 mph and reaching heights of over 70 feet, when striking the coastal regions of Indonesia, India, Africa, and adjacent areas, caused over 250,000 deaths. Volcanic eruptions may also occasionally cause a tsunami with enormous devastation and death. An incredibly severe volcanic eruption occurred on the island of Krakatoa in Indonesia in 1883 that caused a tsunami that killed almost 40,000 inhabitants of coastal regions in neighboring areas.

Because the occurrence of major earthquakes can be detected, it may be possible in the future to alert residents of all coastal regions of the ocean where a major earthquake occurs to evacuate these regions immediately for at least a few hours to avoid an enormous number of deaths and injuries from a tsunami.

In the United States, earthquakes occur mainly on the West Coast, especially in California, but they have occurred as far north as Alaska and rarely in other states (e.g., Missouri, South Carolina, Colorado, Hawaii, and even in the East). No location in the world is entirely free from earthquakes.

Knowledge about the consequences of earthquakes and family emergency planning can be crucial in avoiding or minimizing injuries. Information on how best to prepare and respond to an earthquake is available from the American Red Cross (www.redcross.org), the Federal Emergency Management Agency (www.fema.gov), and the state governor's office.

If you live in an area where earthquakes have occurred, the following have been strongly recommended:

Before an earthquake:

- **Prepare an emergency kit** containing water and food (with a can and bottle opener), flashlights (with extra batteries) and a battery-operated radio (with extra batteries), all necessary medications, and a fire extinguisher. **Be prepared to be self-sufficient for at least 3 days.** Special considerations for older and disabled persons are essential. Keep a fully charged cellular phone available.
- **Designate safe spots** (i.e., under sturdy desks or tables, near interior walls, and away from windows, mirrors, hanging objects, fireplaces, and tall unsecured furniture).
- **Conduct practice drills** so that everyone knows safe locations that are easily accessible during an earthquake, and determine where to reunite if separated. Also, choose an out-of-town relative or friend who can be contacted if necessary.
- **Stability of homes and buildings should be checked and improved** as necessary in all earthquake regions. Fortunately, technology in constructing earthquake-resistant buildings has advanced remarkably and has significantly diminished the risk of building damage and has almost eliminated the collapse of the most recently constructed buildings.

During an earthquake:

- **If indoors, get under a sturdy table or desk, or crouch under a door frame (the latter can be used by an individual confined to a wheel chair). Protect your eyes, head, and neck with your arms and hands.** You may best protect your eyes by pressing your face against your arms. **Stay indoors until the earthquake stops**.
- **If outdoors, get away from buildings, walls, trees, power lines, and steep slopes and drop to the ground.**
- **If driving, pull over and park but avoid parking under an**

overpass, bridge, or near power lines. **Remain in the car until the vibration ends.**

- If in a **crowded public area, do not run for the door but stay in a crouched position and protect your eyes, head, and neck with your arms and hands.**
- If you are **in bed, stay there and protect your head with your arms, hands, and pillows.**

After an earthquake:

- Seek help for any severe injury or other medical problem, but **only in an emergency should you use your vehicle.**
- Immediately report gas leaks, broken electrical wires, and water pipes to your utility companies. **Never light a match if you smell gas, and turn off the gas line if possible.**
- Check your building for damages, and extinguish any fires if possible.
- Always comply with instructions broadcast on your portable radio.
- Remain calm, assist others, and **be prepared for aftershocks** and protect yourself as mentioned previously.
- Do not attempt to cross damaged roads.
- Do not go near downed power lines, and **never** step into water that is in contact with a severed power line as you might be electrocuted.

If you have to leave your residence for any length of time, it is important to leave a note explaining your whereabouts to family members and friends.

Cold Weather

Be aware of the possible harmful effects of exposure to excessive cold. Adequately protecting children, infants, and babies from cold cannot be overemphasized.

1. Frostnip

Inadequate insulation and clothing protection from extreme cold and wind may quickly cause frostnip of the ears, nose, cheeks, chin, tips of fingers, and toes. Shoes or boots that are tight should be avoided, as they can impair the circulation in the feet and aggravate the condition. The skin may become white, pale, or waxy, and because it is painless, it is often unnoticed by the individual. Pressure of a warm hand or blowing hot breath on the area or holding the fingers in the armpits can help restore the circulation and relieve the frostnip. The area should not be rubbed, especially with snow. It should be mentioned that in very cold weather one should never touch or grasp cold metal with an ungloved hand because the skin may become stuck to the metal and cause tearing of the skin when the hand is pulled away. For the same reason, one should never press the face, lips, or tongue against a very cold metal object.

2. Frostbite

Frostbite of the superficial skin is more serious than frostnip, and it may occur rapidly within 10 to 15 minutes with extreme cold exposure. It causes a white, waxy appearance that is firm and numb to the touch. Skiers in particular may be exposed to cold weather with a high wind, especially while riding a chairlift. Adequate face protection (e.g., a ski mask) may be essential to avoid frostbite. **The individual should enter a warm area where the skin can be warmed. However, rubbing should be avoided, as it can cause more tissue injury!** With warming, the area may become bluish or purple and start to ache. Subsequently, the affected area may remain very sensitive to cold and require careful protection whenever the weather is cold and windy. It is reported that **cigarette smoking can increase the occurrence and severity of frostbite, as nicotine causes constriction of blood vessels;** decreased circulation to tissue exposed to cold can aggravate tissue damage caused by frostbite.

Severe frostbite of the deep tissues of the skin and severe cooling of the body are extremely serious conditions. These more commonly occur in hunters, hikers, climbers, and skiers exposed to severe cold, but they may occur in inadequately clothed individuals, alcoholics, and ill or very young or very old and fragile persons exposed to ordinary cold for prolonged periods.

The duration of exposure, temperature, and wind velocity are the three most important factors causing serious injury to the skin or entire body. Wet clothes will further increase the loss of body heat. Tissues are initially cold, pale, and firm, but the injured area may turn purplish or blue and become painful with large blisters or gangrene. These individuals require immediate medical attention, and they should be transported to a hospital as soon as possible. Immersion in very cold water will cause a marked decrease in body temperature that can be rapidly fatal.

3. Winter sports injuries and dangers

It is always so tempting to walk on an ice-covered body of water—**don't do it!** You have no way of being certain that the ice is thick enough to hold your weight. Breaking through the ice and becoming immersed in ice-cold water can also be rapidly fatal, even for those who are not trapped and submerged below the ice and are able to reach the surface where the ice gave way. **Immersion in water at near freezing temperature usually causes unconsciousness and death within 15 minutes.** The efforts of individuals to rescue the victim may result in more persons crashing through the ice and possibly additional fatalities.

It is always absolutely essential to obtain immediate help from the fire department or police. However, if professional assistance is not available, a ladder or board may be placed on the ice and pushed to the victim to provide some support for the victim to pull himself or herself from the water and then receive appropriate treatment.

There are some occasions when ice-covered water may be safe to walk or skate on or to use for "ice fishing." Generally, with prolonged subzero temperatures, ice on a lake becomes thick enough to support considerable weight. However, with a warming trend and with temperatures rising periodically above freezing, walking or skating on the ice should always be avoided. Community officials and the police and fire departments should constantly check ice conditions above water before permitting or preventing its use for recreation. **Always look for and obey signs that warn that ice is thin and dangerous to walk or skate on.**

Hunters, climbers, hikers, and skiers should never explore alone. If a severe injury occurs, the help from companions may be crucial to survival. Neck injuries may be very serious and are best managed by professionals who are knowledgeable about the need for minimizing motion of the neck and prompt transportation to a medical facility. The dangers of becoming lost or buried in an avalanche are well known to most adults, and one should never explore or ski out-of-bounds areas unless authorized by professionals familiar with the terrain.

4. Snow removal

During cold weather, the possible hazard posed by ice or snow accumulation on the roof of cars or trucks should be appreciated. While driving, particularly at a rapid speed, ice can dislodge and may become an "ice missile" that crashes into a closely following vehicle. Severe damage, injuries, and death have sometimes resulted to persons in vehicles struck by the ice. Therefore, it is essential to remove significant amounts of ice from the roof of any vehicle before driving. It is also important to remove large accumulations of snow, as snow may blow off the roof and temporarily interfere with the visibility of a driver in a nearby vehicle. **It is always extremely important to remove deep snow from blocking the exhaust pipe of a vehicle. A blocked exhaust pipe can cause carbon monoxide to accumulate in a stationary vehicle with the**

motor running and the windows closed, and it can cause death or permanent damage to the brain of those in the car.

The danger of overexertion in cold weather, such as shoveling snow, should be recognized, especially by middle-aged and older persons. **Strenuous exercise may result in a heart attack that can be fatal.** Let the younger generation have the pleasure of shoveling snow! **If you use a snowblower, never use your hands to unblock the machine while it is running; always turn off the motor before trying to remove any blocking material.**

For the safety of all, do not cover fire hydrants with snow; they should always be visible and easily accessible to the fire department.

5. Icy pavements

Walking on icy pavements and street crossings is also exceptionally dangerous. Slipping, falling, and sustaining serious fractures or head injuries are not uncommon and are sometimes fatal. **The best way to minimize the chance of falling is to walk very slowly, with a wide base (feet more separated than usual).** Also, boots with treaded rubber soles are less likely to slip on ice than other soles. The old remedy of applying salt to melt ice and/or sand to decrease the chance of slipping will prevent many injuries and sometimes may be lifesaving.

Homeland Security and Terrorism

We all appreciate that the possibility of a terrorist attack in the United States is very real despite efforts of the federal, state, and local governments to strengthen our nation's security. **It is therefore crucial to be "aware and prepare" and follow the advice and recommendations of the U.S. Department of Homeland Security and Department of Health regarding a terrorist attack. The fol-**

lowing information is available in more detail from these government agencies.

Four major types of attack may occur:

1. A **biologic attack** results from a deliberate release of germs that may be inhaled, ingested, or enter through a cut in the skin and cause illness.

2. A **chemical attack** is the deliberate release of toxic gas, liquid, or solid that can poison individuals by contaminating the environment.

3. A **"Dirty Bomb"** spreads harmful radioactive material over an area when common explosives cause the bomb to explode.

4. A **nuclear blast** is an extremely powerful and devastating explosion accompanied by intense light and heat with a severe damaging pressure wave and widespread radioactive material contaminating the air, water, and ground surfaces for miles around.

The possibility of a nuclear attack by a terrorist is very unlikely at this time, but a biologic, chemical, or "Dirty Bomb" attack are distinct possibilities. Other terrorist activity that could have devastating effects would be the explosions caused by (1) bombs on subways, trains, buses, planes, or ships, (2) by suicide bombers in crowded areas, or (3) by rocket-propelled explosive devices aimed at aircraft or other targets. Any of these could cause severe damage and casualties. In addition to the death and injury of many individuals in the area of the explosion, the psychologic and economic impact could be very damaging to Americans and the nation. As we all know, a nuclear explosion could kill and injure an enormous number of persons; however, with proper preparation and management, casualties caused by other terrorist attacks can be limited and relatively small. **In case of a terrorist attack, "above all, stay calm, be patient, and think before you act."**

Planning and common sense can save lives. Preparing for an emergency and having a plan to communicate with family members who may be separated are essential. The decision to remain where you are or to leave that location and travel to another location will depend on the type of attack and the instructions of the government and local administrations. If you are in a location where the surrounding air may be contaminated, it may be necessary to remain indoors and sheltered from the contamination. The U.S. Department of Homeland Security recommends the following:

Staying Put: There are circumstances when staying put and creating a barrier between yourself and potentially contaminated air outside, a process known as "shelter-in-place," can be a matter of survival. Choose an interior room or one with as few windows and doors as possible. Consider precutting plastic sheeting to seal windows, doors and air vents. Each piece should be several inches larger than the space you want to cover so that you can duct tape it flat against the wall. Label each piece with the location of where it fits.

If you see large amounts of debris in the air, or if local authorities say the air is badly contaminated, you may want to "shelter-in-place." Quickly bring your family and pets inside, lock doors, and close windows, air vents and fireplace dampers. Immediately turn off air conditioning, forced air heating systems, exhaust fans and clothes dryers. Take your emergency supplies and go into the room you have designated. Seal all windows, doors and vents. Watch TV, listen to the radio or check the Internet for instructions.

Getting Away: Plan in advance how you will assemble your family and anticipate where you will go. Choose several destinations in different directions so you have options in an emergency. If you have a car, keep at least a half tank of gas in it at all times. Become familiar with alternate routes as well as other means of transportation out of your area. If you do not have a car, plan how you will leave if you have to. Take your emergency supply kit and lock the door behind you. If you believe the air may be contaminated, drive with your windows and vents closed and keep the air conditioning and heater turned off. Listen to the radio for instructions.

At Work and School: Think about the places where your family spends time: school, work and other places you frequent. Talk to your children's schools and your employer about emergency plans. Find out how they will communicate with families during an emergency. If you are an employer, be sure you have an emergency preparedness plan. Review and practice it with your employees. A community working together during an emergency also makes sense. Talk to your neighbors about how you can work together.

The U.S. Department of Homeland Security stresses the importance of first thinking about fresh water, food, and clean air. They recommend at least a 3-day water and food supply (one gallon of water per day for each person and enough canned and dried food for each person, plus a manual can and bottle opener, plastic cups, and eating utensils). For babies and young infants, include bottles with nipples, baby food, formula, disposable diapers, etc. Be prepared to care for older persons and those who are ill or handicapped. Special plans to care for pets should be made, as it must be recognized that pets are not permitted in shelters used for humans. In addition, the following items should be available in a supply kit:

1. A battery-powered radio and extra batteries
2. Flashlight and extra batteries
3. Matches in a waterproof container
4. First-aid kit and a pair of scissors

5. Prescription medicine for those on medication

6. Filter masks that cover the mouth and nose of adults or children

7. Plastic bags for sanitation use if needed

8. Duct tape and heavy-weight garbage bags or plastic sheeting to seal windows and doors, if necessary, to protect from outside air contaminants. Also, air conditioners should be turned off. However, sealing off the air supply can be dangerous and should only be done if officials advise you to do so.

9. If you are living in a cold region, be sure to have adequate warm clothing.

It is important that family members know where emergency supplies and the first-aid kit are kept. Also important phone numbers (e.g., police, fire department, the local health department, Poison Control Center, and an out-of-area family contact) should be available at the home, work place, and school.

It is critical to listen to your radio for important announcements and instructions so that you will know the best procedures to follow to best protect your family and where to go to receive appropriate vaccines and medications. Know which radio stations can supply you with important and current local information.

Family, friends, neighbors, work-place associates, school administrators and teachers, and entire communities should all be prepared to work efficiently and effectively with the police, fire department, the medical profession and care givers, and governmental agencies to minimize the damaging effects of any terrorist attack. Being well prepared can save lives and reduce injury.

For additional and more detailed information, contact your local Department of Health, the U.S. Department of Homeland Security website at www.ready.gov, the Centers for Disease Control and Prevention website at www.cdc.gov, or the American Red Cross at www.redcross.org.

Being prepared to respond properly to a terrorist attack is your best protection.

Avoiding Bites

Rabies

Although adults are aware of the risks of being bitten by dogs, cats, ferrets, or other animals, adults and parents should warn children repeatedly about these risks. Furthermore, **in the event of anyone being bitten, medical attention should always be promptly obtained, and whenever possible, the animal that caused a bite should be placed under observation for development of rabies.** Bites from bats should be taken seriously and treated by a physician, as they also may transmit rabies in their saliva. **Rabies is always fatal but can be prevented by prompt immunization.**

Insects

Efforts should always be implemented to prevent or at least minimize the risk of bites from ticks, mosquitoes, bees, wasps, hornets, yellow jackets, fire ants, spiders, snakes, and scorpions. Never disturb or attempt to remove a hornet's nest if you are unfamiliar with the proper procedures and precautions to prevent being stung. **Those allergic to insects should carry an EpiPen (for injecting adrenaline) that can be used promptly if a sudden allergic reaction occurs after any insect sting.** Stagnant water should always be eliminated, as mosquitoes use this water to breed; chemical sprays are also helpful in destroying mosquitoes.

Mosquitoes can transmit a variety of viruses (e.g., West Nile virus) that can cause brain inflammation and nerve damage, or they can transmit a parasite that causes malaria (very rare in the United States). The bites of some of these insects, spiders, and scorpions may be very painful and may cause severe reactions and even death. **Children should be educated about the importance of avoiding these bites. Medical attention should be sought promptly if a significant reaction occurs after any bite.**

Snakes

Snakes are usually found in southern states, especially from Florida to California; however, poisonous snakes inhabit the entire United States, except Maine, Alaska, and Hawaii. Most snakes live on the ground in the mountains, forests, or deserts, but some thrive in rivers, streams, wetlands, and swamps where they may bite swimmers or those wading in these areas; some hang from trees and may bite those passing by. **One should never disturb or handle wild, possibly poisonous snakes, and it is very important to avoid stepping or sitting on a snake or putting a hand into an area where a snake may not be seen.** Leather boots extending above the ankles may protect persons from being bitten if a snake is stepped on. When walking in the dark, making a loud noise may make snakes move away from your path; however, it is wise to use a flashlight. Most bites occur in individuals walking in rural areas in sandals or bare feet at night without any light. Rattlesnakes usually cause a rattling sound, especially when disturbed, but this does not always occur; they account for most poisonous snakebites and are responsible for almost all snakebite deaths in the United States. **If an individual is bitten, the bite should not be cut or sucked, and a tourniquet should not be applied to an arm or leg. It is best to apply a light bandage. If the wound is on an arm or leg, the bitten extremity should be immobilized and medical attention at a hospital should be ob-**

tained as soon as possible. Administration of snake antivenin may occasionally be indicated.

Scorpions

Scorpions in the United States are usually found west of the Mississippi River, especially in Arizona and southern California. They often live in crevices and burrows or under woodpiles, rocks, or buildings where it is cool, and they inhabit the desert, grasslands, forests, plains, and caves. Scorpions may enter houses, if the doors are left open, and get into shoes, clothing, bedding, bathtubs and sinks in search of water. **Doors should always be closed, and shoes, clothing, and bedding should be examined and shaken to be sure scorpions are not present**. The venom of some scorpions may cause severe pain, swelling, and other serious manifestations; however, death is rare, and an antivenin treatment is available for severe cases.

Ticks and Lyme Disease

Ticks may transmit a number of diseases, including Lyme disease. Lyme disease is caused by the bite of a tick infected with a spirochete germ that lives in some rodents, other warm-blooded animals, and birds. Because adult ticks preferentially feed on deer, the increasing deer population in some regions, including residential areas, enhances the chance of infection. Deer are not infected by the spirochete, but they can carry ticks that are infected and can transmit the disease to humans. Lyme disease has become increasingly common in many parts of the United States, especially in northeastern states from Massachusetts to Maryland and in Minnesota and Wisconsin; however, cases have been reported in 49 states. Most cases occur during the spring and summer months when ticks are frequently found in moist regions in high grass and wooded areas. Cases have occurred particularly in association with hiking, hunting, and camping. Persons can be reinfected with Lyme disease, but the disease cannot be transmitted from one human to another.

It is important to recall ways to protect yourself and your family from becoming infected. For those exposed to a tick-infested area, the Lyme Disease Foundation and the Centers for Disease Control and Prevention recommend:

1. **Wear light-colored clothing** so that ticks are easy to see and can be brushed off.

2. **Tuck pants into socks and your shirt into your pants** to prevent ticks from reaching the skin. When hiking, **stay in the middle of trails.** Try to **avoid contact with tall grass and bushes,** and **avoid sitting on the ground.** At home, it is wise to **remove leafy litter, wood, and garbage and to mow grass frequently. Letting grass dry thoroughly between waterings will help eliminate ticks, as they need moist habitats to live.** Very high fences (at least 10 feet high) can help prevent deer from entering residential properties.

3. **Use repellents containing DEET (available in the United States as Ultrathon and "Off!") on the skin (*but not on the hands or near the eyes*).** It should be applied according to Environmental Protection Agency guidelines to reduce the possibility of toxicity. One application is effective for only about 1.5 hours; thus, it should be repeatedly applied to be effective as a repellent. Wash off repellents when you return inside.

4. Use the insecticide permethrin (Permanone) on outer clothing only. This is nontoxic to humans, nonstaining, and odorless, and it remains effective for several days. **When used together, DEET (applied to exposed skin) and permethrin (applied to outer clothing) provide nearly 100% protection from ticks, mosquitoes, chiggers, and fleas.**

5. **After coming indoors, examine your body and your children for ticks.** Especially check the groin, navel, armpits, behind knees and ears, and between toes, and have a companion check your back; children should be checked at least once daily and every few hours in areas heavily infested with ticks. Young ticks may be very small, about the size of the head of a pin, and may be missed unless the entire body is carefully examined. However, some adult ticks may be the size of a raisin. Ticks on clothing can be easily killed by washing the clothes or placing them in the dryer for 30 minutes.

6. **Remove ticks as soon as possible** because transmission of the spirochete germ that causes the disease is less likely if a tick is removed within 36 to 48 hours after attachment.

7. It is best to remove the tick immediately with tweezers by grasping the tick as close as possible to the skin and pulling gently without crushing or puncturing the body of the tick because it may contain infectious fluid. After removal, any head parts remaining in the skin should be removed like a splinter and whenever possible, all parts should be placed in a tightly closed container and checked by a local or state health department laboratory for evidence of the Lyme germ. If the germ is identified, treatment is indicated. After removal, disinfect the skin, and wash the hands with soap and water.

8. **See a physician if an expanding circular red rash develops at the site of a tick bite** (60% to 80% of persons infected will develop this rash at the site of the bite within a few days to a month) **and/or if the person develops other manifestations** (e.g., fever, headache, fatigue, muscle and joint aches, nerve or brain inflammation, enlarged lymph nodes, stiff neck, conjunctivitis, or abnormal heart function). A tick bite is painless, and there is usually no history of a bite. Check with your physician to be sure that testing for Lyme disease is done by a reliable laboratory. Unreliable results are sometimes reported in the United States and elsewhere in the world.

Because Lyme disease may infect some animals, a veterinarian should be consulted if your dog, cat, horse, or farm animals become ill. Animals should be kept out of tick-infested areas as much as possible. They should be checked daily, and any ticks should be removed promptly. A veterinarian should be consulted about the use of tick repellents and the best ways to minimize Lyme disease infections in animals.

Consult your physician and the Lyme Disease Foundation (1-800-886-5963) for additional information about Lyme disease and how best to protect your family from becoming infected. Treatment with certain antibiotics is usually very effective in eliminating the disease.

Although Lyme disease is the most common illness transmitted by ticks in the United States, it must be appreciated that ticks can transmit a variety of diseases. Therefore, when in a tick-infested area, it is important to make every effort to avoid tick bites, but it is essential to consult a physician if a child or adult develops a fever, headache, chills, sweats, muscle pains, a rash, fatigue, nausea, vomiting, diarrhea, loss of appetite, or rarely anemia, sometimes accompanied by jaundice (yellowish color of the skin).

Avoiding Bear Attacks

When hiking or hunting in some parts of the United States, Canada, and Mexico, it is important to know how to minimize the possibility of a bear attack. In some states, bears even enter suburban populated areas. Black bears inhabit 32 of the United States, whereas grizzly bears are rare in North America outside of Alaska and Canada. Black bears are not uncommon—especially in the Shenandoah Valley, Appalachian Trail, the Great Smoky Mountains, Yellowstone, and the Grand Teton National Parks, Georgia, parts of Pennsylvania and New Jersey. They are especially active around dawn and dusk.

Bears are shy and rarely attack humans; however, they have good eyesight and an excellent capacity to smell scents miles away, and they are always looking for food. They hibernate during the winter but are active at other times, and the highest rates of human attacks occur in the fall and during the hunting season. They sleep in grassy meadows, dense brush, near fallen trees, and near logs. Most of the following are strongly recommended by the Forest Department and professional personnel who are responsible for supervising, preserving, and protecting our national parks:

- **Always hike or hunt with a partner or in a group so that assistance can be given to anyone injured or taken ill.** Bears are less likely to approach several people than a single person. Be alert to surroundings and don't focus entirely on hunting game. **Wherever permitted it is important to have a high-powered rifle immediately available at all times.**
- **Keep campsites clean at all times—scent of food, garbage, feces, urine, etc. can attract bears. Even change clothes if they smell—especially if there is any odor of food.**
- **It is extremely important to keep food (also cooking utensils, drinks, toothpaste, soap, and any scented items) in bear-proof containers or in a sturdy bag hung on a strong branch of a tree at least 10 feet above the ground and at least 6 feet from the tree trunk.** The bag should be hung a considerable distance (at least 100 yards) from your campsite. This will prevent a bear from reaching your food and will minimize the chance of a bear intruding on your campsite. If you have a vehicle nearby, food can be kept in the trunk of the car. Cook and eat meals away from your tent or shelter. In suburban areas where bears often intrude, it is recommended that garbage be placed in bear-proof containers.
- **Never feed bears or leave food behind for them, since this will increase the risk to you and others who follow.**
- If you smell a dead animal, do not investigate.

- **Don't shoot a bear unless it attacks.** A wounded bear can be very dangerous to you and others.
- If you encounter a bear, it will probably run away, unless you have food nearby. **If the bear remains, you should back away slowly, watching the bear but not making eye contact. Do not run away, since you can't run as fast as a bear and do not play dead. If a bear approaches, dropping a hat or some garment (but not anything with food) may cause the bear to stop and examine what you have dropped—giving you time to move slowly away, but never running. If a bear attacks and you don't have a gun, then you should throw stones at the bear's head, use sticks or fists if necessary to defend yourself. Strike bears on the nose or eyes if possible. Assuming a "cannon ball" position may end the bear attack.**
- **Avoid startling bears, but it is helpful to make noises—talking, singing, shouting or clapping hands. However, shrill or high-pitched noises and bells may arouse and attract bears. If you see a bear, never approach to take a photo. Calmly leave the area, talking loudly so that the bear knows you are leaving.**
- Keep children with you at all times, and where dogs are permitted keep them on a leash and under control.
- **Never come between a bear and its cubs.**
- Bear repellents (e.g., pepper spray) only work at close range and may anger a bear and further endanger you.
- Always have flashlights for use at night, and, in case of an emergency, a cell phone should be carried. A satellite cell phone may be needed in some areas where there are mountains and valleys.

Polar bears in North America inhabit Alaska and parts of Northwest Canada (i.e., the Yukon territory). These very large bears, with their white fur, blend into the background of ice which makes it easy for them to sneak up on their prey. Polar bears do not usually attack humans, but they may appear suddenly "out of nowhere." **If someone is alone, they are more likely to be attacked. Therefore, it is very important to remain in groups when in polar bear territory. Several powerful rifles are needed in case a bear attacks.**

Although grizzly bears have caused the greatest number of fatal bear attacks on humans, polar bears may occasionally view humans as prey. Young adult and female polar bears with cubs are particularly dangerous. **The same precautions to minimize bear attacks by black and grizzly bears (mentioned previously) should be taken with polar bears.**

Be alert, keep a clean camp, reduce food and garbage smells to a very minimum. Keep away from food sources, and keep food out of the reach of polar bears (at least 12 feet above the ground). If a bear approaches, get into a nearby vehicle, if present, and drive away. If, despite making noise and backing away without making eye contact, a polar bear continues to approach, it is probably best to shoot the bear—at least several times to make sure the bear is killed. A wounded bear can be especially violent and dangerous. However, only rare instances have been recorded of humans being killed by polar bears.

Health Emergencies

Blood Clots

Development of blood clots in the legs or elsewhere can be a serous risk, as sometimes these clots may travel to the lungs and cause death. Therefore, it is strongly recommended that individuals who have ever had blood clots in their legs should frequently move about every 1 or 2 hours on a long plane flight. Long car trips should be interrupted at least every few hours to take a short walk. If there are no contraindications, taking a regular aspirin before the trip will provide additional safety by decreasing the tendency of the blood to clot. The sudden occurrence of shortness of breath, pain in the chest when taking a breath, or coughing up blood may be manifestations of a blood clot in the lung and requires immediate medical attention by a physician.

Heart Attacks

Immediately contact your physician if any pain or sensation of pressure or tightness occurs in your chest, especially if it persists for more than 20 to 30 minutes. The discomfort may be mild or moderate, but sometimes it is very severe and extends into the back, neck, jaw, stomach, or down the arms; it may be accompanied by shortness of breath, sweating, nausea, and vomiting. With these manifestations, there is a strong possibility that you are having a **heart attack** that is caused by a blockage of a blood vessel in the heart. **Call 911 immediately for ambulance and medical assistance, and then take one regular aspirin (unless you are allergic to aspirin or are taking blood thinners). Try to contact your physician.** To be more effective, a drug that dissolves a clot (a "clot buster") blocking an artery in the heart should be given within 1 hour of the onset of a heart attack. **Do not delay getting medical help. Acting immediately may save your life and limit heart damage.**

Strokes

It is very important to recognize symptoms of a stroke (sometimes called a "brain attack"). Stroke results from a sudden brain injury caused by inadequate blood supply, 80% resulting from a blocked artery and 20% caused by a hemorrhage from a ruptured artery. Brain damage may be large or minimal, following a small temporary blockage, that is a TIA (a "ministroke"). The most common stroke symptoms are:

- **Sudden numbness or weakness** of the face, arm, or leg, especially on one side of the body.
- **Sudden confusion and difficulty understanding or speaking**—speech may be "slurred."
- **Sudden blurred or decreased ability to see**, especially in one eye.
- **Sudden dizziness and loss of balance, coordination, and difficulty walking**.
- **Sudden severe headache**, unlike any previous headaches, with no known cause.

Symptoms of a TIA are similar to a stroke except symptoms disappear within minutes to hours.

If any of these manifestations occur, it is extremely important to call 911 immediately so that a prompt diagnosis and appropriate treatment can be administered in a hospital as soon as possible. A delay of more than 3 hours in treating a patient with a stroke caused by a blood clot or hemorrhage may prevent the ability to open successfully a blocked brain artery or limit the amount of bleeding. Appropriate treatment without delay can reduce mortality and disability.

The following are recommendations that may help to prevent a stroke:

- Lower an elevated blood pressure to normal.
- Stop smoking—especially if you are taking birth control pills containing estrogen and progesterone.
- Become physically active and lose excess weight.
- Lower elevated harmful cholesterol (LDL).
- If you have diabetes, carefully control your blood sugar.
- Avoid excess consumption of alcohol—no more than two drinks for men and one drink for women.
- Take one baby aspirin daily, if there is no medical reason not to use it; check with your doctor.

Preventive Measures For Your Health

Immunization

Influenza Vaccination

Yearly influenza (flu) vaccination is safe and often effective in preventing or minimizing influenza infections. Influenza is a serious disease that causes about 36,000 deaths each year in the Unites States. A flu shot is recommended each year (preferably in October or early November), especially for

- All children 6 to 23 months old
- Individuals over 65 years old
- Those with chronic diseases
- Those with HIV/AIDS or other conditions and those with a weak immune system
- Women who are pregnant during the flu season (usually November to March)
- Physicians, nurses, or anyone coming in close contact with people at risk for developing influenza
- Residents of nursing homes and long-term care facilities
- Persons 6 months to 18 years old on prolonged aspirin treatment, as they may develop another serious condition (Reye's syndrome) if they get influenza.

Flu vaccine should not be given to individuals who are allergic to eggs or who have had a serious reaction to a former flu vaccination. Also, anyone who has had the rare disease called Guillain-Barré should not be vaccinated. Finally, those with a fever or who are temporarily ill should postpone vaccination until they have recovered.

Pneumococcal Vaccination

Pneumococcal vaccination is indicated in persons 65 years of age or older, and it should be repeated in 5 years or more frequently in persons 80 years or older. Vaccination is **also indicated in persons with chronic diseases, including those with a weakened immune system** (e.g., HIV/AIDS infection and those with no spleen). Pneumococcal disease causes more than 40,000 deaths in the United States annually, and more than half of these may be preventable with vaccination. Vaccination should not be administered to those with a history of allergies or severe reactions to other vaccinations. In individuals with fever or an acute illness, vaccination should not be given until the patient recovers. Revaccination every five years is not indicated, except in the elderly or those who lack a spleen or have certain chronic diseases.

Tetanus

Although the importance of immunizing children is well recognized, adults often fail to obtain the necessary booster (reimmunization) shots every 10 years to protect themselves against a tetanus infection.

Influenza and pneumococcal vaccinations are extremely safe and only very rarely cause any significant reaction, and they can be given at the same time. For further information about vaccinations, a doctor should be consulted.

A physician should be consulted regarding immunizations and disease precautions before travel to areas where infectious diseases are common and sanitation is poor.

Eye and Ear Safety

Shatterproof glasses or protective goggles should be worn when playing sports involving small firm balls that may strike and injure the eye. Similarly **protection of the eyes** is important when operating machinery that may eject particles that can injure the eyes. Protection from contact with caustic chemicals that can damage the eyes must always be observed. The need to **protect the ears from recurrent loud noise** is not always appreciated, especially by teenagers. Repeated exposure to loud noises caused by motors or gun firing or loud music can impair hearing permanently.

Health Screenings

Cancer

In addition to occasional checkups regarding blood pressure, blood sugar, blood fats, and routine eye and dental examinations, **adults should consult physicians about indications and appropriate methods of screening for skin, breast, colon, cervical, ovarian, prostate, testicular, and lung cancers and tuberculosis**. Screening is crucial, as these conditions usually cause no symptoms when they first develop. A full examination of the skin by a dermatologist is rarely done; however, early detection of a melanoma may be life-saving. A yearly skin examination is very worthwhile, especially in those exposed to lots of sun. Women should learn how they can best examine their breasts. Men should check their scrotum for any lumps or swelling (normally one testicle is larger than the other). Any abnormalities or changes discovered by self-examination (at least monthly) should be immediately reported to a physician.

Persons with a family history of colon polyps or cancer, breast, or prostate cancer are at increased risk for developing these tumors and should be screened periodically. **Cigarette smokers are at a very high risk for developing lung cancers, and therefore, they should probably have a special chest X-ray (CAT scan) each year if they have smoked more than one pack of cigarettes daily for 20 or more years.**

Blood Cholesterol

Furthermore, it is recommended that adolescent children with a family history of early heart disease, or a parent with high cholesterol, or whose parents' histories are unknown, have their blood cholesterol determined. About 50% of adults have elevated harmful cholesterol in their blood. Therefore, it is advisable to get a blood test to determine if you have any abnormalities. An easy rule to remember is "100, 50, 150"; that is, LDL (bad cholesterol) should be 100 mg or less. HDL (good cholesterol) should be 50 mg or more, and triglycerides (another bad fat) should be 150 mg or less. If any of these are abnormal, consult a physician; if they are normal, you may wait about 5 years before rechecking these levels.

Bone Density

About 10 million American adults have osteoporosis, and 80% are women. Women 65 years or older and men 70 years or older should be screened for bone thinning. However, **women and men 50 years or older with risk factors for osteoporosis (e.g., a family history of osteoporosis, a small or thin body size, a cigarette smoker, a previous history of fractures, or taking corticosteroid medication) should especially be screened for bone thinning**. Osteoporosis usually causes no symptoms before it results in fractures and damage to the bones in the spine. The importance of efforts to prevent or identify disease in an early stage of development cannot be overemphasized.

Minimizing Health Care Errors

It is a shocking fact that up to 100,000 deaths are caused each year in the United States by errors mainly of doctors and nurses. This has been called an "epidemic of medical mistakes," which is exposed in a riveting account by Drs. Robert M. Wachter and Kaveh G. Shojania in their book *Internal Bleeding*. Despite these horrific mistakes, the authors point out that "modern medicine has a dark side only because its light shines so brightly." Certainly, the quality of medicine in the United States is the best in the world, and it is likely that mistakes by doctors and nurses occur as often or more often in other nations as they do in the United States.

Efforts are constantly being made by hospitals to improve health care and to minimize mistakes; however, because no person or system is infallible, a number of medical and surgical errors are bound to occur. Drs. Wachter and Shojania, professors at one of America's leading medical schools and two of the foremost authorities on healthcare errors, have skillfully outlined key ways of reducing the number of mistakes that may occur and improving your medical care and that of your family. The following suggestions and comments by the authors (with minor modification) will increase your involvement with your doctor and other healthcare personnel:

1. **Make an effort to understand the name, action, and dose of your medications.** It is better for doctors to avoid abbreviations when writing prescriptions. **Be sure you can read a prescription before leaving the doctor's office.** This will be helpful to your pharmacist, as a number of drugs sound alike and look alike. **Ask your doctor and pharmacist whether there are any risks of harmful drug interactions.**

2. **Check whether your doctor is board certified in his or her specialty.** Certification indicates a certain level of competence that may be superior to those who are not certified.

3. **Keep medications in their original containers, which should have their name and dose.** If you change dose, be sure to use the new container. **Bring all of your medications (including alternative medications) to your doctor's office on each visit, and be sure your doctor has a list of all your drug allergies.**

4. **If you are having an operation on a symmetrical body part (eye, ear, arm, leg, kidney, lung,) be sure that the correct part of the body is the one being prepared for operation.** As a double precaution to avoid the risk of error, the side to be operated can be marked.

5. **Ask whether you should receive any treatments to prevent blood clots, infections, or heart problems.**

6. **Check the expertise and experience of the physician who will perform the surgery or procedure on you at an institution (http://www.leapfroggroup.org/consumer-intro2.htm).**

7. **Before you get a medication, transfusion, imaging study (X-ray, MRI, etc.), or a procedure, make sure the nurse, phlebotomist, and other hospital personnel check your wristband and/or ask your name and date of birth.**

8. **Before being taken off the floor for a procedure, ask what the procedure is, and make sure that you understand where you are going and why. Be sure you are the correct patient.**

9. **Be sure that your family members' contact information is available to the hospital or nursing home personnel.**

10. **Before being transferred to another floor in a hospital or from one institution to another, be sure that your doctor knows whether you have a urinary catheter.** Prolonged use of a catheter poses a risk of urinary track infection, and thus, it should be removed if its continued use is unnecessary.

11. **Check with your doctor and nursing staff regarding your blood type to make sure that you are receiving properly matched blood before being transfused. Also check to be sure you are receiving a properly matched tissue transplant.**

12. **Indicate in your chart whether you wish doctors to attempt to resuscitate you if your heart stops beating or you stop breathing.** This is a delicate subject that should be discussed with your family and doctor. Many patients with serious incurable disease may not want to be resuscitated and wish to have "do not resuscitate (DNR)" appear in their chart.

Large medical centers, especially those attached to medical schools, have many physicians with outstanding expertise and a depth of experience that make them more qualified than most physicians in small hospitals. It is believed that the onsite presence of physicians who coordinate patients' care in the intensive care units (ICUs) results in a better outcome and improves patient safety.

The patient-to-nurse ratio is important on the medical and surgical wards because it is reported that a ratio of 6 to 7 patients for every nurse is associated with a higher risk of errors. Furthermore, it is reported that if 25% to 30% of care is being given by licensed practical nurses rather than RNs (registered nurses) there is a higher risk of errors. All nurses in the ICU should be RNs, and it is recommended that there should be one RN for every two patients. It is reported that hospitals with a higher percentage of RNs with bachelor's degrees had lower postoperative mortality rates.

Finally, there is evidence that clinical pharmacists on the wards and available to help patients understand and organize their medication, particularly at the time of discharge, improves safety.

For the detailed understanding of the medical mistakes that occur in our nation and how best to minimize these errors, *Internal Bleeding* is very highly recommended. **It seems quite clear that if patients play a more active role in their care and are also better informed about the management of their illness, the risk of medical and surgical errors will be substantially reduced.**

First Aid Courses

CPR

It is strongly urged that adults learn how to perform CPR (cardiopulmonary resuscitation) on a person who has stopped breathing or whose heart has stopped beating. When and how to administer electroshock if the heart has stopped should also be learned, especially because equipment to administer electroshock may be readily available in locations used by large numbers of people. Proper administration of these procedures requires training by professionals who are knowledgeable in these resuscitation techniques. (American Red Cross, www.redcross.org).

Heimlich Maneuvers

The **Heimlich maneuvers** may be learned from instructions on manikins to demonstrate the proper techniques of performing these procedures to dislodge food (often a piece of meat) that is stuck in the throat and is causing airway obstruction. These individuals usually point to their neck and are in obvious distress and unable to speak. Prompt action is necessary and can be life saving.

Summary

This list suggests only some of the causes of serious and often preventable injuries. Most important, however, is that parents follow good judgment and assume the responsibility for doing their utmost to anticipate the possible occurrence of injuries before they happen by intervening with effective preventive measures. **It is said that good judgment comes from experience and that experience comes from bad judgment. Perhaps these few warnings and suggestions may help to prevent both bad judgment and tragic experiences.** Periodic family discussions regarding safety measures (including fire drills) to prevent injuries can be particularly informative and may save lives. The importance of child safety cannot be overemphasized, and we must constantly strive to educate our children and make every effort to maximize their safety.

RISKS of Inadequate Sleep

Many live in a sleep-deprived condition that can significantly impair job performance, academic achievement, excellence in sports activities, judgment, decision making, reflexes, and dexterity involved in driving a car or handling potentially dangerous equipment. According to the National Sleep Foundation, drowsiness and fatigue play a role in 100,000 car collisions each year in the United States. Excess alcohol consumption or the use of illicit drugs, of course, will markedly increase automobile as well as other injuries related to fatigue.

In her recent book, *Adolescent Sleep Patterns*, Dr. Mary Carskadon, who is engaged in sleep research at Brown University, indicates that inadequate sleep may have serious consequences, especially on the mental and physical health of adolescents. She observes that some "students may be in school, but their brains are at home on their pillows." **Teenagers seem to function best if they obtain 9 to 10 hours of sleep each night; most adults may require about 8 hours of sleep for optimal performance. Concentration, learning ability, and memory are diminished by sleep deprivation, and feelings of anxiety, depression, irritability, combativeness, and hostility may appear with marked increases in aggressive behavior and violence.** As Dr. Carskadon pointed out, sleep loss in animals also is associated with "marked increases in aggressive behavior and violence."

There is some evidence in humans and animals that inadequate sleep may impair the immune system, which is important in combating infections and preventing some malignant tumors. Adults appear more likely to have a heart attack if they are sleep deprived. Furthermore, as mentioned previously, it appears that getting 6 hours or less of sleep daily is associated with increased obesity. A hormone called leptin was recently found to decrease markedly in individuals who were allowed to get only 4 hours of sleep each night. The deficiency of leptin may then cause an effect on the brain that increases appetite.

About 4% of adult Americans have sleep apnea, which is a periodic cessation of breathing during sleep, usually caused by airway obstruction in the back of the mouth and upper airway tube. Sleep apnea is significantly more common in middle-aged and older men who are overweight and especially in obese and hypertensive individuals. Rarely, obese children or those with enlarged tonsils or adenoids may have sleep apnea. Loud snoring, restlessness, and interrupted sleep almost always accompany sleep apnea, and often persons with this condition remain tired and drowsy throughout the day. **Episodes of apnea may be accompanied by development of hypertension, stroke, heart attack, and premature death. These individuals often suffer from sleep deprivation that cannot be cured by lifestyle modification.** Medical or surgical treatment and weight reduction (if indicated) are required to manage this potentially serious sleep disorder.

Doctors and sleep experts agree that parents should play a stronger role in ensuring that their teenagers get adequate sleep. This obviously may be a difficult and demanding task. **However, setting a specific bedtime, for example, 10 P.M., on school nights is essential; the importance of limiting time on the television, telephone, and computer is crucial.** Adequate sleep should continue during the weekends, but excess ("binge") sleep on the weekends should be avoided. Significant deviation from an adequate sleep routine can disrupt the success of a healthy sleep pattern and the accompanying sense of well-being derived from such a program. Teenagers will often resist and object to any sleep curfew or time restriction on the use of TV, telephone, or computer; however, they should recognize that parents who make these demands are doing so to improve the health and happiness of their children. Studies indicate that most sleep disturbances in children and teenagers occurred in those with TVs in their bedrooms, especially in those who fell asleep watching TV. It always should be stressed that nothing is more powerful than example in influencing others. Parents who avoid excessive use of the TV, telephone, and computer and who routinely retire at a reasonable time (e.g., by 11 P.M.) usually will find it easier to influence their children to do so. **The key, however, to ensure success in establishing a healthy sleep program for teenagers is for parents to be firm, persistent, and consistent in their demands.**

Although the sleep of some adults who drink coffee regularly may not be disturbed by consuming caffeine (which stimulates the brain) at dinnertime, children and teenagers should avoid beverages and foods containing this stimulant. Some medications contain other stimulants that can disrupt sleep. Excessive excitement and strenuous exercise should be avoided near bedtime, as they may interfere with the ability to fall asleep. Alcohol consumption and heavy eating shortly before retiring may disrupt sleep and aggravate sleep apnea. It is important for some adults to appreciate that naps during the day can interfere with a sound sleep at night. Deep breathing, a soft, soothing background sound (e.g., of the ocean) or music, and being trained in various ways to relax and minimize anxiety may help those suffering from insomnia. It is recommended that a comfortable, medium–firm mattress be used and room temperature be about 68°F, and light rather than heavy pajamas are preferable. The room should be very quiet and without disturbing light. Furthermore, it is best to use a dim light if toilet use is necessary during the night, as a bright light can disturb sleep.

Occasional, painful leg cramps may occur at night which awaken persons who are sleeping. It is usually necessary to get out of bed and walk a few steps to relieve the pain. Curling your toes upward rather than downward may also relieve a cramp in your calf muscle. Keeping your legs warm and wearing socks may help prevent foot and leg cramps, and sometimes an antihistamine medication may prove helpful; however, first consult your doctor.

It has been reported that about 12 million Americans experience what Dr. John Winkelman, a faculty member at Harvard Medical School and Director of the Sleep Health Center, describes as "creepy-crawly, jittery, gnawing sensations that worsen at night". These sensations occur in the calves or feet and sometimes in the arms. There is usually an irresistible urge to move the affected limbs. Inactivity makes the sensations worse; however, they are relieved by movement. Furthermore, the restless leg syndrome (RLS) can disrupt sleep. This periodic movement disorder may sometimes be related to iron deficiency anemia or kidney failure. Dr. Winkelman states that drugs that increase brain dopamine (a nerve hormone) have been remarkably effective in treating individuals with RLS. Caffeine, pregnancy, and lack of sleep often make the condition worse. Dr. Carl Hunt, Director of the National Center on Sleep Disorders Research in Bethesda, Maryland recommends that you consult your physician if you are having problems sleeping, since "there are serious medical consequences of ignoring poor sleep".

In general, medication to induce and maintain sleep is not recommended; however, when necessary, consumption of Tylenol or Tylenol PM may be helpful in inducing sleep. The decision to use stronger medications should be left to the judgment of a physician, as some drugs used repeatedly may cause addiction. In general, children should not be given sleeping medication.

Risks of Inadequate Sleep

Stress RISKS

In our pressurized modern society, stress (mental or emotional tension) and anxiety have become increasingly common and seriously interfere with the quality of our lives and that of our family and associates. Dr. Bruce S. McEwen (at Rockefeller University in New York City), a co-author of a recent book, *The End of Stress As We Know It*, predicts that "by 2020, depression will be the second leading cause of disease in this country," second only to disease of the heart and blood vessels.

Factors said to contribute to chronic stress are:

- Conflicts at home or at work
- Social isolation
- Overworking
- Sleep deprivation
- Lack of exercise
- Overeating
- Excess fat in the diet
- Smoking
- Excess alcohol consumption
- Economic problems
- Fears of war and terrorism
- Procrastination (delay of things that should be done)

Dr. McEwen emphasized the importance of maintaining social ties with friends and family (i.e., social support), getting adequate sleep, eating a balanced, nutritious diet, and regular, moderate exercise. Most important is his advice that "a healthy lifestyle is the best way to reduce stress." A healthy lifestyle will usually give one a sense of control and a positive outlook.

Finally, regarding anxieties over terrorism, Dr. Lewis Goldfrank, head of emergency medicine at Bellevue Hospital and New York University Medical Center, has his emergency room very well equipped and prepared for a terror attack. He does not recommend vaccinating most doctors or the public for smallpox because the chance of a serious reaction is more likely than being harmed by weaponized smallpox. Dr. Goldfrank suggests that we be more focused on public health by improving our lifestyle. When he was a featured speaker at an International Congress on Disaster Psychiatry in Washington, DC, he was expected to talk about emergency management of bioterrorism. Instead, he emphasized the serious dangers of obesity and drunk driving, which are far more likely and preventable than nuclear, biological, or chemical attacks.

In the event of a chemical, biological, or nuclear attack, it is crucial that everyone be able to follow instructions and guidance by government agencies, police and fire departments, and medical centers. It is absolutely essential to have a battery-operated radio (with extra batteries) immediately available at all times.

Concluding Remarks

In a book of uncommon and profound wisdom entitled *A Mind at a Time*, Dr. Mel Levine, a pediatrician and perhaps America's top learning expert, shows how every child can succeed. He is deeply committed to helping children develop successfully. **The essence of this remarkable book is that all children have different minds and different abilities and that far too much emphasis has been placed on academic achievement with little effort to discover and develop specific abilities and talents.** Too often, poor students are viewed as intellectually inferior and failures. These children feel humiliated and embarrassed by their inability to perform well in school. A sense of inferiority and a lack of self-confidence can lead to feelings of helplessness and hopelessness, which can generate internal rage. As a consequence, these children may become severely depressed, delinquent, often they drop out of school, and resort to illicit drug use, violence, and crime.

As Dr. Levine pointed out so well, "Everyone is intelligent in one way or another." He urges, "Parents, teachers, and policy makers to recognize how many kinds of young minds there are and to realize we need to meet their learning needs and strengthen their strengths and in so doing preserve their hopes for the future." Discovering and then developing special abilities of children, teenagers, and adults can give self-confidence, self-respect, self-esteem, and a sense of self-fulfillment that can add pride, dignity, and direction to their lives. **Encouragement is vital in developing self-esteem and an optimistic view of one's potential for reaching future goals. In addition, a healthful lifestyle is also essential for optimal development of body and mind.**

A healthy lifestyle is extremely important not only for physical health, but also for emotional stability and self-esteem. It often is the key to success and happiness. Obesity, sedentary lifestyle, alcoholism, addiction to smoking, illicit drug use, acquisition of sexually transmitted disease, and chronic stress can impair health, self-esteem, and quality of life. Furthermore, lack of self-esteem and a sense of insecurity can be responsible for some of these unhealthy lifestyles. **The importance that self-esteem can play in all our lives, but especially in the development of children, cannot be overstated. The present and future success and the health of this nation depend mainly on the lifestyles of our society and the character of our youth!**

The VITAL (Values Initiative Teaching About Lifestyle) program is aimed at the *prevention* of unhealthy lifestyles and their health consequences. The key to the success of this program is that, at appropriate ages, it teaches children and teenagers about the risks of unhealthy lifestyles *before* unhealthy lifestyles are acquired. To be most effective, parents must participate with their children in the VITAL program. An established unhealthy lifestyle in many adults and teenagers can be difficult if not impossible to remedy. **Therefore, improvements in prevention strategies are worth every possible effort. Never starting an unhealthy lifestyle is easier than having to stop it.**

Because the future of our nation depends to a large degree on the character of our youth, it is our responsibility and duty to make every effort to help our society and our children adhere to a healthy lifestyle and find meaning, success, and happiness in their lives.

By improving our lifestyle and habits, we can surely reach a "higher, warmer, and purer" quality of life. "The human soul longs for things, higher, warmer, and purer, than those offered by today's mass living habits" (from a Harvard Commencement Address in 1978 by Alexander Solzhenitsyn). **Improving lifestyle is always possible.** Let us remember to "Dwell in Possibility," as Emily Dickinson suggests. **A healthy lifestyle is surely the best road to a longer and better life.**

Acknowledgments

It is *pure delight* to thank those wonderful associates and friends who have given so much of their time and talent to improve the quality of this book.

For extraordinary and exceptional editorial assistance and for concisely clarifying the text and improving its structure:

> Paul Piazza   Associate Headmaster and Former Chairman of the English Department, St. Albans School, Washington, DC

> Richard Ruge   Tax consultant, PriceWaterhouseCoopers; Former Managing Editor of the *Harvard Crimson*

For very significantly improving the content and presentation of the text:

> Porter F. Fleming, Esq.   Patent Lawyer, New York, NY

> Thomas E. Forschner   Director, Lyme Disease Foundation

> Lewis Goldfrank, MD   Physician, Head Emergency Medicine, Bellevue Hospital, New York, NY
> Chairman, Department of Emergency Medicine, New York University Medical Center, New York, NY

> Ruth Johnston   Research Assistant, National Hypertension Association, New York, NY

> Alla Krayko   Secretary and assistant administrator, National Hypertension Association, New York, NY

> Kristie J. Lancaster, PhD, RD   Assistant Professor, Department of Nutrition, Food Studies and Public Health, New York University, NY

Charles S. Manger   Real Estate Business Executive, New York, NY

Jules N. Manger, MD   Physician, Head Emergency Medicine, Concord Hospital, NH

Lynn S. Manger   Founder and Emeritus Chairman, Parents In Action; Advisory Board, National Association for Drug Abuse Problems; Former member of New York City Youth Board, New York, NY. Co-director of Values Initiative Teaching About Lifestyle (VITAL)

Stewart S. Manger   Fine Arts and Design, New York, NY

William M. Manger, Jr.   Regional Administrator, Northeast and Caribbean, U.S. Small Business Administration, New York, NY

Jennifer K. Nelson, MS, RD   Director of Clinical Dietetics, Mayo Clinic, Rochester, MN

Shlomoh Simchon, PhD   Physiologist, Co-Director of Research, National Hypertension Association, New York, NY

Siri Sirichanvimol, MS, RD   Former Clinical Manager of Nutrition, New York University Medical Center, New York, NY

Clifford M. Yonce   Vice President, Goldman Sachs Trustee, National Hypertension Association, VITAL Program, New York, NY

For helpful consultation and guidance regarding publication:

Christopher Davis   Publisher, Jones and Bartlett Publishers, Sudbury, MA

Kate Hennessy   Associate Production Editor, Jones and Bartlett Publishers, Sudbury, MA

Gillian Steelfisher   Director of Strategy, Cogent Research, Boston, MA

Muir N. Weissinger   Author, St. Augustine, FL

Gale M. Wood   Cardiovascular Research Foundation and Author, New York, NY

For translating a short version of this book into Spanish:

Sherry Rusher   Chair, Foreign Language Department, St. Albans School, Washington, DC

Commentaries

"I commend this superb book to readers of all ages who wish to achieve a healthy lifestyle."

D. Nelson Adams, Esq.
(Former Managing Partner, Davis, Polk & Wardwell Law Firm
New York, NY)

"Dr. Manger's book articulates the basic tenets for good health clearly and simply. This book is a must read for all persons interested in health and well-being."

Henry Barbey
(Director, The New York Center for Coaching, Inc.
Adjunct Professor, New York University)

"You challenge each of us to take the control we *do* have. You've provided a well-presented and surely informed overview for many things we can know about and act upon to increase our prospects for good health."

Dr. Ralph Blair
(Liturgist, The City Church, New York, NY)

"This is a book about life, not in the fast lane, not in the dull lane, but in the lane of productivity, happiness, and good karma. It has been written not by a 'feel good, mind doctor,' not by a huckster with something to sell, but by a physician who cares about people and who gives easily understood advice on recognizing the serious pitfalls of everyday living and what exactly to do about them. Read it, follow its advice, and you will be a better person."

John Braasch, MD, PhD
(Former Chairman of Surgical Department, Lahey Clinic
Assistant Clinical Professor of Surgery, Harvard Medical
School, Boston, MA)

"Really good and will be extremely helpful to the audience this is intended for. The DASH diet is terrific."

Kelly D. Brownell, MD
(Director, Yale University Center for Eating and Weight Disorders
New Haven, CT)

"Excellent."

Denis A. Cortese, MD
(President and Chief Executive Officer,
Mayo Foundation, Rochester, MN)

"It is wonderfully provocative: every chapter is of interest to (and important to) everybody. [Dr. Manger has] done it very impressively and professionally. Bravo!"

Honorable Walter J.P. Curley
(Former Ambassador to Ireland and France
New York, NY)

"Kudos! Remarkably understandable for the lay public. Extremely thorough and easy to read besides the fact that it is interesting in its presentation."

Isabelle B. Dayton
(Artist, Vero Beach, FL)

"A very comprehensive work dealing with many cogent issues. It is a must read for both families everywhere and practitioners of medicine. You bring out some too infrequently discussed issues with helpful advice for all."

John T. Dayton, MD
(Physician, Vero Beach, FL)

Commentaries

231

"Seems solid and well expressed and likely to be of benefit to parents and teenagers. A wonderful job in preparing this material."

Andrew G. Frantz, MD
(Professor of Medicine and Associate Dean of Admissions,
Columbia University,
College of Physicians and Surgeons, New York, NY)

"It would seem essential for us to accomplish all the issues that [Dr. Manger is] working on in an effective manner to make society safer and better. Congratulations on your work."

Lewis Goldfrank, MD
(Chairman, Department of Emergency Medicine,
NYU School of Medicine,
Director, Department of Emergency Medicine,
Bellevue Hospital, New York, NY)

"Here it is! A stepping stone to reach your personal best."

Catherine Grant
(Map librarian, Central Intelligence, retired
Washington, DC)

"A wonderful, practical guide to healthy living that can be easily read and understood by all."

Eric Grant
(Director, Community Affairs and Contributions,
The Washington Post)

"Dr. William Manger is a true humanitarian and patriot, and his deep concern for humankind inspired him to create a perfect manual to enhance the quality of life for all who are willing to adhere to its guidelines."

Skip Grant
(Former Director of Athletics and The Skip Grant Program,
St. Albans School, Washington, DC)

"Dr. Manger has clearly and factually outlined measures to ensure good health. I would advise all to read this book, especially parents raising children. Good health habits should start early in life."

Robert S. Gordon, MD, FACP
(Associate Clinical Professor of Medicine, Yale University,
Woodbridge, CT)

"Readers of the book will in fact live longer and live better if they heed its advice. It addresses a wide variety of important every day health issues and does so in an authoritative yet readable manner."

Francis J. Haddy, MD, PhD
(NASA Peer Review Services
Former President, American Society of Physiology
Washington, DC)

"It is well written, interesting, informative, and comprehensive. I learned a lot from reading it. The book should serve as a resource for intelligent, well-educated, and well-motivated parents, as well as for teachers, social workers, psychologists, nurses, and other health professionals."

Theresa B. Haddy, MD
(Pediatrician, Rochester, MN)

"Great—and so important. It should be required reading for parents and teachers of all our youngsters growing up on junk food and vending machine drinks."

Mildred Hulse, MS
(Formerly Research Associate,
NYU Medical Center, New York, NY)

"This is excellent—providing practical information in a readable manner that should be helpful to almost everyone."

Norman M. Kaplan, MD
(Professor of Internal Medicine, University of Texas, Dallas, TX)

"Splendid, inspiriting, hugely informative, crystal-clear prose and impassionate."

The late Michael Kenyon
(Author and professor, Southampton College,
Southampton, NY)

"Well written, clear, accurate, and interesting."

Jeffrey P. Koplan, MD, MPH,
(Former Director, Centers for Disease Control and Prevention
Currently, Vice President for Academic Health Affairs
Atlanta, GA)

"Excellent [book]. I think it will really impact positively on the lives and lifestyles of many children."

Mel D. Levine, MD
(Director, Clinical Center for the Study of Development and
Learning
University of North Carolina at Chapel Hill, NC)

"Useful, informative, and very easy to read. My reactions are very positive."

Ralph I. Lopez, MD
(Clinical Associate Professor of Pediatrics,
Cornell Medical College, New York, NY)

"Dr. Manger's years of experience provides good sound advice and encouragement to make healthy adjustments to our lifestyles. Thank you for providing such expert guidance and the inspiration to carry out these important principles to help so many parents and children. With his educational and research accomplishments, commitment to family, and ethical and considerate treatment of other people, Dr. William Manger is certainly an extremely credible mentor for a healthy lifestyle."

Charles C. Manger, III, MD
(Ophthalmologist and CEO, Saddleback Eye Center
Laguna, California) and Mrs. Charles C. Manger, III

"I believe it belongs on the same shelf with the Bible, the dictionary, and the encyclopedia."

Marion Martin Manger
(Mother, grandmother, and great-grandmother
Dallas, TX)

"An excellent idea and a great presentation. A most useful road map for preventive measures for good health. Dr. Manger covers the field totally in easy-to-understand language and easy-to-appreciate examples. The most important theme is that you can take control of so many aspects of your health."

Alexander A. Minno, MD
(Physician, Pittsburgh, PA)
Mrs. Alexander A. Minno
(Lawyer, Pittsburgh, PA)

"Most impressed—very well put together."

N. Stephen Ober, MD, MBA
(President, Beyond Genomics, Inc., Waltham, MA)

"Provides impressive and useful information to help Americans protect and improve their health. I like the clear, positive messages which are energetic."

Edward J. Roccella, PhD, MPH
(Coordinator, National High Blood Pressure Education Program
Bethesda, MD)

"An excellent summary of the many lifestyle issues that we should be thinking about as we make choices for ourselves and our children. It certainly is a timely book as we recognize the health consequences of ubiquitous fast food choices, the lack of exercise in most people's lives because of the competition of TV and the Internet, and the incredibly fast pace of life that leaves less time for sleep and social interactions."

Suzanne H. Rodgers, PhD
(Consultant in Ergonomics, Rochester, NY)

"His book is truly a work that needs to be heard by those who wish to experience life to the max. His experience will motivate and inspire any reader."

Dr. Robert A. Schuller
(Minister, The Crystal Cathedral
Garden Grove, CA)

"A superbly informative health guide! Excellent reading for parents! Through this book, Dr. Manger has provided a great service to those who care about the future of our country—our children!"

Dr. Robert H. Schuller
(Minister, The Crystal Cathedral
Garden Grove, CA)

"Dr. Manger's book is a transforming, practical gallop that spells out in everyday language the nuts and bolts, do's and don't's for preventing maladies and mishaps, and how to achieve optimal health and feelings of well-being. *Our Greatest Threats* should become an indispensable compendium-treat for readers, their families, and those yet to come."

Berthold E. Schwarz, MD
(Psychiatrist, Vero Beach, FL)

"This is the best information regarding the 'heart smart' or 'best diet' for the lay person that I have ever seen. I think it is outstanding."

James Sowers, MD, FACE, FACP
(Associate Dean of Clinical Research
Professor of Medicine, Physiology, and Pharmacology
Director, the University of Missouri
Diabetes and Cardiovascular Center
Columbia, MO)

"I believe this book can make a profound difference to the quality of life for millions of Americans and beyond." (This is) "a serious guidebook for all of us to read, study, inwardly digest, and live by, day-by-day."

Alexandra Stoddard
(Author, designer, and contemporary philosopher)

"A masterpiece—brilliantly done—the most thorough, to the point life guideline for all of us, from birth to the grave."

Jean F. Waters
(Director, Fitnastics, Rochester, MN)

"Admirably clear and direct, free of jargon, even though [Dr. Manger goes] to some pains—which is also admirable—to give the medical background of each piece of advice. Many of the things [he says] are *worth* hearing twice."

Tom Wolfe
(Author, *The Right Stuff* and *Bonfire of the Vanities*)
New York, NY)

Commentaries

Index

A Mind at a Time (Levine), 222
Abdominal obesity, 24
Adolescent Sleep Patterns (Carskadon), 212
Adolescents
    alcohol consumption among, 86, 123
    automobile safety, 134
    and danger of being hit by a car, 142
    fire safety, 150
    gun safety, 154
    illicit drug use by, 111, 115, 118, 122, 123–124
    overweight and obese, 14
    safe swimming practices, 144
    and sexually transmitted diseases, 129–130
    sleep deprivation, 212, 214
    smoking and, 97–98, 99
    VITAL program, 223
Aerobic exercise, 79
Agatston, Arthur, 51, 54
AIDS/HIV
    illicit drug use and, 112, 115, 121
    pneumococcal vaccination for patients with, 203
    as sexually transmitted diseases, 128–129, 130, 131
Alcohol cessation/alcohol withdrawal, 90–91
Alcohol consumption, 4–5, 85–91
    and boating safety, 143
    driving while intoxicated, 134–135, 139–140
    and inability to fall asleep, 214
    smoking and alcoholism, 98
    weight gain and, 29, 64
Alcoholics Anonymous (AA), 91
American Academy of Pediatrics, 33
American Automobile Association (AAA), 138
American Diabetes Association, 54

American Heart Association, 32, 43, 58
American Medical Association, 32
American Red Cross, 180
Amphetamine, 114
Amyl nitrite, 119
Androstenedione, 122
Anorexia nervosa, 4
"Apple-shaped" body type, obesity and, 24
Archives of Family Medicine, 25
Arsenic exposure, 171–172
Asbestos exposure, 170–171
Athletes
    marathon runners and salt consumption, 72
    use of ephedra, 32
    use of steroids, 122
    winter sports injuries and dangers, 184–185
Atkins diet, 42, 51–52
Atkins, Robert, 51, 54
Automobile safety, 134–141

Barbiturates, 120
Bariatric surgery, 32, 66
BC bud, 112
Bear attacks, avoiding, 196–199
Bechler, Steve, 32
Beta blockers, 82, 83
Betel nuts, 118
Bicycle safety, 141–142
Binge drinking, 86
Biologic attack, 187
Bites, avoiding, 191–196
Blood cholesterol screening, 204–205
Blood clots, development of, 199
Bloom, Stephen, 10
Boating/sailing safety, 142–144
Body mass index (BMI), 12–14, 17, 66
Body weight, determining ideal, 11–14

Bone density screening, 205
Bulimia, 4
Bupropion, 106
Burgess, George H., 145–146

Calcium, dietary, consumption of
    vitamin D and, 37
Caloric requirements
    alcohol consumption and caloric
        intake, 90
    to maintain a healthy weight,
        58–61, 62
    physical activity and reduced
        caloric intake, 82
Cancer screening, 204
Carbon monoxide, 152–153
Cars, automobile safety, 134–141
Carskadon, Mary, 212
Center for Science in the Public
    Interest (CSPI), 55, 71, 74
Centers for Disease Control and
    Prevention, 10, 194
Chemical attack, 187
Chewing tobacco, 99
Child Safety Protection Act, 159
Child safety seats, 140–141
Children
    arsenic exposure, 171–172
    boating safety, 142–143
    caffeine and inability to fall asleep,
        214
    clothing safety, 161
    and danger of being hit by a car,
        142
    dangers of electric shock, 155
    determination of BMI in, 14
    and dietary choices, 27–28
    discovering special abilities of, 222
    driving with, 140–141
    exercise intensity for, 80
    fire safety, 150, 151
    food-borne illnesses, 155
    food promotion marketing

    strategies directed at, 15
    gun safety, 154
    and a healthy lifestyle, 25, 223
    hypertension in obese, 17
    and lack of physical activity and
        exercise, 76, 77–78
    and lead poisoning, 168, 169
    and mercury poisoning, 167–168
    mold/fungi exposure, 172
    obesity in, 14, 15, 76, 77
    operating tools and machinery
        around, 154
    pedophiles, 161–163
    safe swimming practices, 144
    safety for, 159–163, 209
    smoking and, 97, 98
    sunburn protection for, 148
    swimming pool safety, 146–147
    television and video viewing by,
        15, 76
    toy safety, 159–161
    VITAL program, 6–7, 223
    window bars and safety gates for,
        154
Chlamydia, 128
Cholesterol
    bad cholesterol (LDL), 39, 40, 42,
        79, 95
    blood cholesterol screening,
        204–205
    good cholesterol (HDL), 41, 79,
        95
    in metabolic syndrome, 19–20
Cigar smoking, 94, 95
Cigarette smoking, 4, 93–101
    asbestos exposure and, 170
    home fire deaths and, 150,
        151–152
    lung cancer and, 204
    quitting smoking, 98–99, 103–107
    weight gain and, 64
Clothing safety, children and, 161
Cocaine, 114, 116

Codeine, 121
Coffee and tea consumption
 caffeine and inability to fall asleep, 214
 weight gain and, 29, 63–64
Cold sensitivity, 166
Cold weather exposure, 182–186
Compulsive eating, 31
Condoms, for protection from STDs, 130, 131
Contaminated water, swimming in, 147
CPR, 208–209
Crank (drug), 116
Crash diets, 38–39, 50–51
Creatine, 123
Crisis, definition of, 10

Date rape drugs, 119–120
Death
 alcohol-related traffic deaths, 86–87
 car-crash deaths, 134–135
 choking deaths in children, 160
 home fire deaths, 150, 151–152
 hurricane-related deaths, 174–175
 smoking-related deaths, 94, 98
Department of Agriculture, U.S., 157, 159
Department of Health and Human Services, U.S., 157, 171, 186
Department of Homeland Security, U.S., 186–191
Dextromethorphan, 121
DHEAs, 123
Diabetes, obesity and, 14, 17, 23
Diet and nutrition
 the best eating plan, 35–66
 selecting a healthy diet, 26
Dietary Approaches to Stop Hypertension (DASH) diet, 43–47, 55, 56–58, 61, 73
Dietary supplements
 containing ephedra, 32–33

herbal and plant products, 33
Dirty bombs, 187
Diseases
 attributable to obesity, 10, 17, 18–20, 30–31, 33
 from smoking, 94–95, 96–97
Diuretics, 68
Drug Enforcement Administration, U.S., 123
Drugs
 alcohol and, 91
 antihypertensive medications and alcohol, 91
 antihypertensive medications and exercise, 82–83
 for obesity, 65
Drugs, illicit
 driving under the influence of, 134–135, 139–140
 hallucinogens, 113–114
 inhalants, 118–119
 marijuana, 110–113
 opiates, 120–121
 sedatives, 119–120
 steroids, creatine, DHEAs, 122–123
 stimulants, 114–118
 use of, 123–126
Drunk driving, 86–87

Ear safety, 203–204
Earthquakes/tsunamis, 179–182
Eating disorders, 4
Eating healthy, strategies for, 47–50
Ecstasy, 114, 117, 123
Electric shock, 155
Electrocution, from lightning, 172–173
Environmental factors, and its role in weight gain and obesity, 11, 16–17
Environmental hazards, 167–172
Environmental Protection Agency, U.S., 169, 171

Ephedra, 32–33
Ephedrine, 32
Exercise. *See* Physical activity and exercise
Eye safety, 203–204

Fad diets, 38–39, 50–51
Falls
    falling on icy pavements, 186
    older adults and protection against, 163–166
Fat, dietary, 16, 39–40
    body shapes and, 24
    guidelines for, 30
    high blood fats, 24
    monounsaturated fats, 41–42
    polyunsaturated fats, 42
    saturated fats, 40
    trans-fats (trans-fatty acids), 39, 41
Federal Emergency Management Agency (FEMA), 180
Fire safety, 150–152
First aid courses, 208–209
Floods/hurricanes, 173–177
Flu vaccination, 202, 203
Fluids consumption, weight gain and, 15, 16, 28–29, 63–64
Focus—A Practical Parenting Guide (NYC-Parents In Action), 125–126
Food and Drug Administration (FDA), 32, 41, 53, 159
Food-borne illnesses, 155–156
Food industry
    fast-food restaurants and obesity crisis, 15–16, 26–28
    food marketing strategies, 15, 16
    salt consumption and, 69, 70, 71
Food labels, 39, 41, 69
Food Politics (M. Nestle), 15
Food portions, super-sized, 27–28, 61
Food preparation

fire safety and, 151
    safe, 155–159
Foot cramps, 214
Friedman, Jeffrey, 10–11
Frostbite, 183–184
Frostnip, 183
Fungus exposure, 172

Gas leaks and fumes, 153
Genetic abnormalities, obesity and, 11, 16, 26
Genital herpes, 128
Genital warts, 128
GHB (gamma-hydroxybutyrate), 119
Goldfrank, Lewis, 218–219
Gonorrhea, 128
Guns and pistols, 154–155

Hallucinogens, 113–114
Health care errors, minimizing, 205–208
Health emergencies, 199–205
    preventive measures for your health, 202–205
Health screenings, 204–205
Healthy lifestyle
    children and a, 25
    establishing a, 6
    importance of a, 25, 222–223
    motivation and achieving a, 5

Heart attacks, 200
    smoking and, 97
Heart disease
    obesity and, 17
    smoking and, 96, 97, 98
Heart function, exercise and its benefits for, 79–80
Heart rate
    during exercise, 82–83
    smoking and, 96
Heat sensitivity, 166
Height/weight standards, 11–12, 13

Heimlich maneuvers, 209
Helmets, protective, 140, 141
Hepatitis B, 128
Herbal and plant products, 33
    herbal teas, 29
    use of dangerous herbs, 123
Heroin, 121
High blood pressure. *See*
    Hypertension
Hippocrates, 65
HIV. *See* AIDS/HIV
Home safety, 150–155
Homeland security and terrorism,
    186–191
Human papilloma virus (HPV),
    128
Hunt, Carl, 215
Hurricanes/floods, 173–177
Hypertension
    alcohol consumption and, 89–90
    Dietary Approaches to Stop
        Hypertension (DASH) diet,
        43–47, 55, 56–58, 61, 73
    obesity and, 17, 21–23
    salt consumption and, 68–69, 70,
        72
    smoking and, 96, 97
    weight lifting and, 81

Icy, wet, snow-covered roads
    driving on, 136–137
    walking on icy pavements, 186
Ideal body weight (IBW),
    determining, 59
Immunization, 202–203
Influenza vaccination, 202, 203
Inhalants, 118–119
Insect bites, 191–192
Institute of Medicine, 69
Internal Bleeding (Wachter and
    Shojania), 205–207
Iron, dietary, consumption of, 39
Isometrics, 81

Jacobsen, Mark, 33
Junk food, 15

Keep Off the Grass (Nahas), 112
Ketamine, 119, 120
Khat, 117–118
Klonopin, 120
Knives and sharp instruments, 153
Koop, C. Everett, 11
Koplan, Jeffrey, 10, 16

"Larding of America," 14
Lead poisoning, 168–170
Leg cramps, 214
Lenfant, Claude, 69
Leptin, 10, 212
Levine, Mel, 222
Life expectancy, obesity and, 14
Lifestyle
    changing your, 2-3
    importance of a healthy, 5, 6, 25,
        222–223
Lightning, 172–173
Lopez, Ralph I., 110
Low-carbohydrate diets, 42, 51–52
LSD (lysergic acid diethylamide),
    113
Lung disease, smoking and, 97, 98
Lyme disease, 193–196
Lyme Disease Foundation, 194, 196

Ma huang, 32–33
Malignant melanoma, 149–150
Marijuana, 110–113, 120, 123
Marijuana and Medicine (Nahas),
    112
Mayo Clinic Healthy Weight
    Pyramid, 57
McEwen, Bruce S., 218
Men
    body shape and waist
        circumference in, 24
    caloric requirements for, 58–59

determining ideal weight for,
11–12
obesity in American, 14
Mercury poisoning, 167–168
Mescaline, 113
Metabolic syndrome, obesity and,
19–20
Methadone, 121
Methamphetamine, 114–115
Minority groups, food promotion
marketing strategies directed
at, 15
Mold/fungi exposure, 172
Morbid obesity, 13, 31–32, 66
Morphine, 120
Motivation
and achieving a healthy lifestyle, 5
and quitting smoking, 104
and weight loss, 25
Motorcycle safety, 141
Motorized bicycle safety, 141–142

Nahas, Gabriel G., 112
Narcotics Anonymous (NA), 121
National Academy of Sciences, 55
National Cancer Institute, 43, 58
National Center on Addiction and
Drug Substance Abuse, 125
National Center on Sleep Disorders
Research, 215
National Football League (NFL),
32
National High Blood Pressure
Education Program, 43, 58, 69,
74
National Highway Traffic Safety
Administration, 136
National Institutes of Health, 10
National Sleep Foundation, 212
Nestle, Marion, 15
Net carb, 53
New York Times, 33
Nicotine, 95

nicotine chewing gum, 106
nicotine transdermal patches, 106
Niland, Frank, 137–138
Nuclear blasts, 187

Obesity crisis, 3–4, 9–34
Older adults
food-borne illnesses, 155
safety of, 163–166
Opiates, 120–121
Opium, 120
Orlistat (Xenical), 65
Ornish, Dean, 51
Ornish diet, 53
Osteoporosis, 79, 205
Overweight and obesity crisis, 3–4,
9–34

Passive smoking, 96–97
PCP ("angel dust"), 110, 111,
113–114
"Pear-shaped" body type, obesity
and, 24
Pedometer, using a, 26
Pedophiles, 161–163
Pelvic inflammatory disease (PID),
128
Phencyclidine (PCP), 110, 111,
113–114
Phenylpropanolamine, 32
Physical activity and exercise, 75–84
weight gain, obesity, and lack of,
16, 26
weight loss and, 56, 64–65
Pipe smoking, 94, 95
Pistols and guns, 154–155
Pneumococcal vaccination,
202–203
Poisonings, 167
Pritikin diet, 53–54, 55
Pritikin, Nathan, 53
Pritikin, Robert, 51, 53
Protein

Atkins diet, 42, 51–52
diet and, 42
Psilocybin, 113, 114
Public schools
decrease/elimination of physical
education in, 77
food consumption and obesity
crisis in, 16
obesity prevention programs, 34
sex education in, 129
sports programs, 78
Pyramid, for DASH diet, 57, 58

Quaaludes, 120

Rabies, 191
Restless leg syndrome (RLS), 215
Road safety, 134–142
Rohypnol ("roofies"), 119–120
Roosevelt, Franklin D., 22–23
Rosenthal, Jennifer, 33

Safety and injury prevention
avoiding bear attacks, 196–199
avoiding bites, 191–196
environmental hazards, 167–172
first aid courses, 208–209
health emergencies, 199–205
Homeland security and terrorism,
186–191
minimizing health care errors,
205–208
safe food preparation, 155–159
safety at home, 150–155
safety for children, 159–163
safety in the sun, 147–150
safety of older people, 163–166
safety on or in the water, 142–147
safety on the road, 134–142
weather-related hazards, 172–186
Safety gates, 154
Salt consumption, 4, 55, 67–74

Salt sensitivity, 68
Salt substitutes, 71–72
Satcher, David, 33
Schweitzer, Albert, 25
Scorpions, 193
Sears, Barry, 51, 54
Second-hand smoke, 95
Sedatives, 119–120
Sedentary lifestyle
moderate exercise for sedentary
persons, 78–79
obesity and, 10, 11, 15
Sexual perversions, pedophiles,
161–163
Sexually transmitted diseases
(STDs), 127–131
Shark attacks, 145–146
Sharp instruments, 153
Shojania, Kaveh G., 205–207
Sibutramine (Meridia), 65
Sleep
inadequate, 211–215
weight gain and, 65–66
Sleep apnea, 213
Smoke alarms, 150
Smokeless tobacco, 99
Smoking. See Cigarette smoking
Snacking, weight gain and, 61–63
Snake bites, 192–193
Snow removal, 185–186
Snuff, 99
Sodium chloride (table salt), 68
Soft drinks, weight gain and
consumption of, 15, 16, 28–29,
63–64
Solzhenitsyn, Alexander, 223
South Beach Diet, 54
Soy foods, 42
Sports
marathon runners and salt
consumption, 72
use of ephedra, 32

use of steroids, 122
winter sports injuries and dangers, 184–185
Steroids, 122
Steward, H. Leighton, 51, 55
Stimulants, 114–116
Stomach bypass surgery, 32, 66
Stress, 217–219
Strokes, 200–201
"Sugar Busters" eating plan, 55
Sun, safety in the, 147–150
Sunburns, 147–148
Swimming, diving, and surfing, safety measures for, 144–145
Swimming pool safety, 146–147
Syphilis, 128

Teen Health Book: A Parent's Guide to Adolescent Health and Well-Being, The (Lopez), 110
Teens. See Adolescents
Terrorism, 186–191, 218–219
Tetanus (lock jaw), 153, 203
Tetrahydrocannabinol (THC), 110–111
The End of Stress As We Know It (McEwen), 218
TIA (ministroke), 200, 201
Ticks, 193–196
Tools and machinery, 154
Tornadoes, 177–178
Toy safety, 159–161
Triglycerides
lowering bad cholesterol and, 39, 42
in metabolic syndrome, 19
Tsunamis, 179–182
Twelve Key Guiding Principles for Parents (NYC—Parents In Action), 125–126

Usnic acid, 33

Vanovski, Jack and Susan, 10
Vegetarian diets, 55
VITAL (Values Initiative Teaching About Lifestyle) program, 6–7, 223
Vitamins and minerals, consumption of adequate, 37–38
Volumetric diet, 56

Wachter, Robert M., 205–207
Water consumption, 63, 72
Water safety, 142–147
Weather-related hazards, 172–186
driving during strong winds, 136
Weight bearing exercises, 79, 81–82
Weight lifting, 79, 81–82
Weight loss
eating disorders, 4
tips on losing weight, 50–66
Weight-loss programs, 34
as a medical expense, 26
Weight-regulating hormone, 10
Weight standards
average weight of Americans, 11, 14
determining ideal weight, 11–14
Weight Watchers, 50
Wellbutrin, 106
Welles, Orson, 25
West, Mae, 29
Whippet, 119
Window bars and safety gates, 154
Winkelman, John, 215
Women
body shape and waist circumference in, 24
caloric requirements for, 58–59
determining ideal weight for, 11–12
obesity in American, 14
pregnancy and food-borne illnesses, 155, 156

pregnancy and mercury poisoning,
   167–168
pregnancy and obesity, 39
sexually transmitted diseases, 128
smoking and birth control pills,
   95

Yancopoulos, George, 10

Zone Diet, 54–55
Zyban, 106

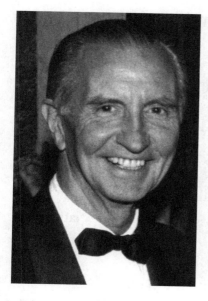

William M. Manger, MD, PhD, is a clinical professor of medicine at New York University Medical Center and former lecturer in medicine at Columbia Medical Center. He is the founder and chairman of the National Hypertension Association and founder and director of the VITAL (Values Initiative Teaching About Lifestyle) program to combat the obesity crisis in the United States. He and his wife are committed to preventing obesity in young children by teaching healthy nutrition and appropriate physical activity through the VITAL program. He also continues to see patients and to conduct research in hypertension.

Dr. Manger received his BS from Yale University, his MD from Columbia's College of Physicians and Surgeons, and his PhD from the University of Minnesota. While a Fellow at the Mayo Clinic, he received the Mayo Alumni Award for Meritorious Research, and in 1992 he received the Mayo Foundation Alumnus Award "in recognition of his exceptional contributions in hypertension for having achieved national and international distinction in research, medical practice, and education and for practicing the high principles which are recognized as exemplary of the founders of the Mayo Clinic and Mayo Foundation."

Dr. Manger and his wife have four children and three grandchildren, and they live in New York City.

Photo Credits for the DASH Pyramid

Bottles of oil: © Photodisc

Stick of butter: Courtesy of Renee Comet/National Cancer
Institute

Container of yogurt: Courtesy of Renee Comet/National Cancer
Institute

Different types of cheeses: © Photos.com

Pitcher of milk with glass: © LiquidLibrary

Strawberry frozen yogurt: Courtesy of Renee Comet/National
Cancer Institute

Loaf and slices of bread: © Digital Stock

Pastas: © Ingrid E. Stamatson/ShutterStock, Inc.

Bowl of cereal: © Digital Stock

Bowl of oatmeal: © John L. Richbourg/ShutterStock, Inc.

Bowl of eggs: © Digital Stock

Fish: © Digital Stock

Roasted turkey: © Digital Stock

T-bone steak: © Digital Stock

Bowl of nuts: © Photodisc

Pecans: © Photodisc

Variety of vegetables: © Photodisc

Beans: © Photodisc

Variety of fruits: © Photodisc

Oranges with orange juice: © Tihis/ShutterStock, Inc.

Green apples: © Photodisc

Stack of cookies: © Samantha Grandy/ShutterStock, Inc

Ice cream in glass: © Kenneth Sponsler/ShutterStock, Inc.

Chocolates: © Jessica Bethke/ShutterStock, Inc.